Australian Breastfeeding + Lactation Research and Science Translation Conference 2024

Australian Breastfeeding + Lactation Research and Science Translation Conference 2024

Volume Editors

Zoya Gridneva
Donna T. Geddes
Nicolas L. Taylor
Debra J. Palmer
Ching Tat Lai
Jacki L. McEachran

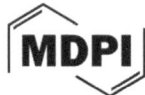

Basel • Beijing • Wuhan • Barcelona • Belgrade • Novi Sad • Cluj • Manchester

Volume Editors

Zoya Gridneva
School of Molecular Sciences
The University of Western Australia
Perth
Australia

Donna T. Geddes
School of Molecular Sciences
The University of Western Australia
Perth
Australia

Nicolas L. Taylor
School of Molecular Sciences
The University of Western Australia
Perth
Australia

Debra J. Palmer
Nutrition in Early Life
Telethon Kids Institute
Perth
Australia

Ching Tat Lai
School of Molecular Sciences
The University of Western Australia
Perth
Australia

Jacki L. McEachran
School of Molecular Sciences
The University of Western Australia
Perth
Australia

Editorial Office
MDPI AG
Grosspeteranlage 5
4052 Basel, Switzerland

This is a reprint of the Proceedings, published open access by the journal *Proceedings* (ISSN 2504-3900), freely accessible at: https://www.mdpi.com/2504-3900/112/1.

For citation purposes, cite each article independently as indicated on the article page online and as indicated below:

Lastname, A.A.; Lastname, B.B. Article Title. *Journal Name* **Year**, *Volume Number*, Page Range.

ISBN 978-3-7258-3603-1 (Hbk)
ISBN 978-3-7258-3604-8 (PDF)
https://doi.org/10.3390/books978-3-7258-3604-8

Cover image courtesy of The University of Western Australia

© 2025 by the authors. Articles in this book are Open Access and distributed under the Creative Commons Attribution (CC BY) license. The book as a whole is distributed by MDPI under the terms and conditions of the Creative Commons Attribution-NonCommercial-NoDerivs (CC BY-NC-ND) license (https://creativecommons.org/licenses/by-nc-nd/4.0/).

Contents

Jacki L. McEachran, Debra J. Palmer, Nicolas L. Taylor, Ashleigh H. Warden, Ching-Tat Lai, Sharon L. Perrella, et al.
Preface and Statement of Peer Review
Reprinted from: *Proceedings* 2025, *112*, 22, https://doi.org/10.3390/proceedings2025112022 . . . 1

Muja A. Gama, Ashleigh H. Warden, Jacki L. McEachran, Demelza J. Ireland, Donna T. Geddes, Sharon L. Perrella and Zoya Gridneva
Breastfeeding Experiences and Milk Production in Mothers of Multiple Birth Infants
Reprinted from: *Proceedings* 2025, *112*, 1, https://doi.org/10.3390/proceedings2025112001 4

Nalini Sirala Jagadeesh, Sangavi Balaji and Rajeswari Singaravelu
Impact of Video-Based Breastfeeding Education on Self-Care Competencies of Postnatal Women
Reprinted from: *Proceedings* 2025, *112*, 2, https://doi.org/10.3390/proceedings2025112002 7

Xuehua Jin, Ching Tat Lai, Sharon L. Perrella, Jacki L. McEachran, Zoya Gridneva and Donna T. Geddes
Hormonal and Macronutrient Profiles in Human Milk Among Women with Low Milk Production
Reprinted from: *Proceedings* 2025, *112*, 3, https://doi.org/10.3390/proceedings2025112003 10

Rajeswari Singaravelu, Temsurenla Jamir and Nalini Sirala Jagadeesh
Effect of Music Intervention on Breast Milk Volume and Stress Among Indian Preterm Mothers
Reprinted from: *Proceedings* 2025, *112*, 4, https://doi.org/10.3390/proceedings2025112004 12

Sofa Rahmannia, Kevin Murray, Gina Arena, Aly Diana and Siobhan Hickling
Distinct Nutrient Sources and Infant Outcomes: Impact of Breastmilk and Complementary Food on Indonesian Infant Growth and Micronutrient Status
Reprinted from: *Proceedings* 2025, *112*, 5, https://doi.org/10.3390/proceedings2025112005 14

Sophie A. Hughes, Zoya Gridneva, Sharon L. Perrella, Donna T. Geddes and Debra J. Palmer
Maternal Factors That Influence the Presence of Food Allergens in Human Milk—A Systematic Review
Reprinted from: *Proceedings* 2025, *112*, 6, https://doi.org/10.3390/proceedings2025112006 16

Zoya Gridneva, Ashleigh H. Warden, Jacki L. McEachran, Sharon L. Perrella, Ching Tat Lai and Donna T. Geddes
Efficacy Assessment of the Breast Shield Size
Reprinted from: *Proceedings* 2025, *112*, 7, https://doi.org/10.3390/proceedings2025112007 18

Zoya Gridneva, Ali S. Cheema, Erika M. van den Dries, Ashleigh H. Warden, Jacki L. McEachran, Sharon L. Perrella, et al.
Breastfeeding Longitudinal Observational Study of Mothers and Kids—BLOSOM Cohort
Reprinted from: *Proceedings* 2025, *112*, 8, https://doi.org/10.3390/proceedings2025112008 20

Zoya Gridneva, Ashleigh H. Warden, Jacki L. McEachran, Sharon L. Perrella, Ching Tat Lai and Donna T. Geddes
Milk Ejections and Milk Flow Patterns During Breast Expression: When to Stop Pumping
Reprinted from: *Proceedings* 2025, *112*, 9, https://doi.org/10.3390/proceedings2025112009 23

Ching Tat Lai, Kim Powell, Yeukai Mangwiro, Tony Frugier, Anna Fedyukova, Jatender Mohal, et al.
GenV: Preservation of Human Milk for Biological Discovery
Reprinted from: *Proceedings* 2025, *112*, 10, https://doi.org/10.3390/proceedings2025112010 . . . 26

Ashleigh H. Warden, Vanessa S. Sakalidis, Jacki L. McEachran, Ching Tat Lai, Sharon L. Perrella, Donna T. Geddes and Zoya Gridneva
Multiple Lactations: Effect of Successive Lactation on Milk Production and Infant Milk Intake
Reprinted from: *Proceedings* **2025**, *112*, 11, https://doi.org/10.3390/proceedings2025112011 . . . 28

Donna T. Geddes, Azhar S. Sindi, Ching Tat Lai, Zoya Gridneva, Gabriela E. Leghi, Mary E. Wlodek, et al.
Impact of Diet on the Maternal and Infant Microbiota
Reprinted from: *Proceedings* **2025**, *112*, 12, https://doi.org/10.3390/proceedings2025112012 . . . 30

Meghan B. Azad
Breastfeeding, Human Milk and Allergic Disease: Findings from the CHILD Cohort Study
Reprinted from: *Proceedings* **2025**, *112*, 13, https://doi.org/10.3390/proceedings2025112013 . . . 33

Jasmine E. Hunt, Philip Vlaskovsky, Ching T. Lai, Sarah G. Abelha, Jacki L. McEachran, Stuart A. Prosser, et al.
Pain Ratings and Pharmacological Pain Management in Australian Breastfeeding Women After a Caesarean Section Birth
Reprinted from: *Proceedings* **2025**, *112*, 14, https://doi.org/10.3390/proceedings2025112014 . . . 36

Sarah G. Abelha, Gloria Cheng, Jacki L. McEachran, Stuart A. Prosser, Diane L. Spatz, Donna T. Geddes and Sharon L. Perrella
Sources and Helpfulness of Breastfeeding Information and Support Accessed by Australian Women Before and After Caesarean Birth
Reprinted from: *Proceedings* **2025**, *112*, 15, https://doi.org/10.3390/proceedings2025112015 . . . 39

Sharon L. Perrella, Jacki L. McEachran, Mary E. Wlodek, Stuart A. Prosser and Donna T. Geddes
Early Feeding Patterns After Pregnancies Complicated by Gestational Diabetes Mellitus
Reprinted from: *Proceedings* **2025**, *112*, 16, https://doi.org/10.3390/proceedings2025112016 . . . 42

Claudia Rich, Jacki L. McEachran, Ashleigh H. Warden, Stuart A. Prosser, Demelza J. Ireland, Donna T. Geddes, et al.
Australian Women's Experiences of Returning to Physical Activity in the Year After Birth
Reprinted from: *Proceedings* **2025**, *112*, 17, https://doi.org/10.3390/proceedings2025112017 . . . 44

Roaa A. Arishi, Ali S. Cheema, Ching T. Lai, Matthew S. Payne, Donna T. Geddes and Lisa F. Stinson
Development of the Breastfed Infant Oral Microbiome over the First Two Years of Life in the BLOSOM Cohort
Reprinted from: *Proceedings* **2025**, *112*, 18, https://doi.org/10.3390/proceedings2025112018 . . . 46

Shanae K. Paratore, Kate A. Buchanan, Sharon L. Perrella and Sara Bayes
Navigating Change: Midwives' Readiness for the Infant Feeding Discussion Page in the West Australian Handheld Pregnancy Record
Reprinted from: *Proceedings* **2025**, *112*, 19, https://doi.org/10.3390/proceedings112010019 48

Ruomei Xu, Mark P. Nicol, Ali S. Cheema, Jacki L. McEachran, Sharon L. Perrella, Zoya Gridneva, et al.
Breastfeeding Characteristics Are Associated with Minor Changes in the Human Milk Microbiome
Reprinted from: *Proceedings* **2025**, *112*, 20, https://doi.org/10.3390/proceedings2025112020 . . . 51

Evangeline G. Bevan, Jacki L. McEachran, Demelza J. Ireland, Stuart A. Prosser, Donna T. Geddes and Sharon L. Perrella
Women's Experiences of Establishing Breastfeeding After Assisted and Unassisted Vaginal Birth
Reprinted from: *Proceedings* **2025**, *112*, 21, https://doi.org/10.3390/proceedings2025112021 . . . **53**

Qiongxiang Lin, Sharon L. Perrella, Ashleigh H. Warden, Cameron W. Evans, Donna T. Geddes, Leon R. Mitoulas, et al.
Nanoscale Imaging of Human Milk Cells
Reprinted from: *Proceedings* **2025**, *112*, 23, https://doi.org/10.3390/proceedings2025112023 . . . **55**

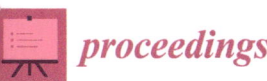

Editorial

Preface and Statement of Peer Review

Jacki L. McEachran [1,2,3,*], Debra J. Palmer [3,4,5], Nicolas L. Taylor [1], Ashleigh H. Warden [1,2,3], Ching-Tat Lai [1,2,3], Sharon L. Perrella [1,2,3], Donna T. Geddes [1,2,3] and Zoya Gridneva [1,2,3]

1. School of Molecular Sciences, The University of Western Australia, Crawley, WA 6009, Australia; nicolas.taylor@uwa.edu.au (N.L.T.); asleigh.warden@uwa.edu.au (A.H.W.); ching-tat.lai@uwa.edu.au (C.-T.L.); sharon.perrella@uwa.edu.au (S.L.P.); donna.geddes@uwa.edu.au (D.T.G.); zoya.gridneva@uwa.edu.au (Z.G.)
2. ABREAST Network, Perth, WA 6000, Australia
3. UWA Centre for Human Lactation Research and Translation, Crawley, WA 6009, Australia; debbie.palmer@uwa.edu.au
4. The Kids Research Institute Australia, The University of Western Australia, Nedlands, WA 6009, Australia
5. School of Medicine, The University of Western Australia, Crawley, WA 6009, Australia
* Correspondence: jacki.mceachran@uwa.edu.au

1. Conference Overview

This publication compiles the proceedings of the ABREAST Conference, held on 15 November 2024 in Perth, Australia. The conference marked another significant milestone in advancing the science and practice of human lactation, bringing together leading experts from around the world to explore innovative research and solutions for improving maternal and infant health.

The ABREAST Conference showcased the latest developments in lactation science, featuring keynote speakers from Australia, Canada, and Denmark. These distinguished experts provided valuable global perspectives, contributing to a diverse and comprehensive examination of the many facets of human lactation. Topics covered included breastfeeding preterm infants in the NICU, improving access to perinatal services for new fathers, the breastfeeding experiences of mothers of multiple birth infants, the human milk microbiome and its role in infant allergies, breastfeeding infants with type 1 diabetes, and initiatives aimed at improving breastfeeding outcomes among urban Western Australian Aboriginal communities through continuous quality improvement efforts. These diverse topics reflect the holistic nature of the conference, which emphasised both the scientific and social dimensions of breastfeeding and lactation.

The ABREAST Network remains dedicated to fostering inclusivity, diversity, passion, and innovation in lactation research. This commitment is evident not only in the range of research topics presented, but also in the network's continued drive to make a meaningful difference in the lives of mothers, infants, and communities worldwide. The ABREAST Conference creates a platform for collaboration, bringing together researchers, clinicians, students, and community stakeholders to exchange knowledge and insights in a dynamic and engaging environment.

This year's conference was once again a resounding success, with 140 total registrations and a strong slate of high-quality research submissions. A total of 22 manuscripts, including those from invited and keynote speakers, were considered for inclusion in the conference proceedings. Of these, 6 manuscripts were accepted for oral presentation and 16 for poster presentation, and 22 manuscripts have been published as part of this volume. This publication will serve as a valuable resource for those seeking to deepen their understanding of human lactation and its critical role in maternal and infant health.

In conclusion, the 2024 ABREAST Conference was another highly successful and impactful event. It reinforced the importance of collaboration, knowledge exchange, and the ongoing advancement of research in the field of human lactation. The conference continues to inspire new research, foster innovation, and support policies that promote breastfeeding and improve maternal and infant health outcomes globally.

2. Conference Committees

2.1. Organising Committee

Mrs. Jacki L. McEachran, The University of Western Australia, Australia.
Dr. Zoya Gridneva, The University of Western Australia, Australia.
Prof. Donna T. Geddes, The University of Western Australia, Australia.
Dr. Sharon L. Perrella, The University of Western Australia, Australia.
Dr. Ching-Tat Lai, The University of Western Australia, Australia.

2.2. Scientific Committee

Dr. Zoya Gridneva, The University of Western Australia, Australia.
Assoc/Prof. Debra J. Palmer, The Kids Research Institute Australia, Australia.
Assoc/Prof. Nicolas L. Taylor, The University of Western Australia, Australia.
Prof. Donna T. Geddes, The University of Western Australia, Australia.
Dr. Ching-Tat Lai, The University of Western Australia, Australia.

2.3. Chairs

Session I: Prof. Donna T. Geddes, The University of Western Australia, Australia.
Session II: Dr Sharon L. Perrella, The University of Western Australia, Australia.
Session III: Assoc/Prof Debbie J. Palmer, The Kids Research Institute Australia, Australia
Session IV: Prof. Donna T. Geddes, The University of Western Australia, Australia.

2.4. Technical Chairs

Dr. Ching-Tat Lai, The University of Western Australia, Australia.
Mrs. Jacki L. McEachran, The University of Western Australia, Australia.

2.5. Registration Chairs

Ms. Ashleigh H. Warden, The University of Western Australia, Australia.
Ms. Sarah G. Abelha, The University of Western Australia, Australia.
Mrs. Jacki L. McEachran, The University of Western Australia, Australia.

2.6. Conference Judges—Student Poster Presentations

Assoc/Prof. Debbie J. Palmer, The Kids Research Institute Australia, Australia.
Prof. Donna T. Geddes, The University of Western Australia, Australia.
Assoc/Prof. Nicolas L. Taylor, The University of Western Australia, Australia.
Dr. Matthew Payne, The University of Western Australia, Australia.
Dr. Leon Mitoulas, Medela AG, Switzerland.
Mr. Phillip Vlaskovski, The University of Western Australia, Australia.

2.7. Editors

Dr. Zoya Gridneva, The University of Western Australia, Australia.
Prof. Donna T. Geddes, The University of Western Australia, Australia.
Dr. Nicolas L. Taylor, The University of Western Australia, Australia.
Assoc/Prof. Debra J. Palmer, The Kids Research Institute Australia, Australia.
Dr. Ching-Tat Lai, The University of Western Australia, Australia.

Mrs. Jacki L. McEachran, The University of Western Australia, Australia.

2.8. Proceedings Compilation Team

Dr. Zoya Gridneva, The University of Western Australia, Australia.
Mrs. Jacki L. McEachran, The University of Western Australia, Australia.

3. Student Prize Winners—Sponsored by Nutrients (MDPI)

Frist Prize—Ms. Jasmine Hunt, The University of Western Australia, Australia.
Second Prize—Ms Claudia Rich, The University of Western Australia, Australia.
Third Prize—Ms Xuehua Jin, The University of Western Australia, Australia.

4. Statement of Peer Review

When submitting conference proceedings to the journal *Proceedings*, the volume's editors notify the publisher that they carried out a peer review of all published papers. Reviews were conducted by expert referees while upholding all the professional and scientific standards expected of the *Proceedings* journal.

- Type of peer review: single-blind.
- Conference submission management system: Email.
- Number of submissions sent for review: 22.
- Number of submissions accepted: 22.
- Acceptance rate (number of submissions accepted/number of submissions received): 100%.
- Average number of reviews per paper: 2.
- Total number of reviewers involved: 5.

Conflicts of Interest: The authors declare no conflict of interest.

Disclaimer/Publisher's Note: The statements, opinions and data contained in all publications are solely those of the individual author(s) and contributor(s) and not of MDPI and/or the editor(s). MDPI and/or the editor(s) disclaim responsibility for any injury to people or property resulting from any ideas, methods, instructions or products referred to in the content.

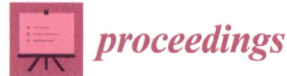
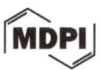

Abstract

Breastfeeding Experiences and Milk Production in Mothers of Multiple Birth Infants †

Muja A. Gama [1,2,3,4], Ashleigh H. Warden [1,2,3], Jacki L. McEachran [1,2,3], Demelza J. Ireland [4], Donna T. Geddes [1,2,3], Sharon L. Perrella [1,2,3] and Zoya Gridneva [1,2,3,*]

1. School of Molecular Sciences, The University of Western Australia, Crawley, WA 6009, Australia; 22898927@student.uwa.edu.au (M.A.G.); ashleigh.warden@uwa.edu.au (A.H.W.); jacki.mceachran@uwa.edu.au (J.L.M.); donna.geddes@uwa.edu.au (D.T.G.); sharon.perrella@uwa.edu.au (S.L.P.)
2. ABREAST Network, Perth, WA 6000, Australia
3. UWA Centre for Human Lactation Research and Translation, Crawley, WA 6009, Australia
4. School of Biomedical Sciences, The University of Western Australia, Crawley, WA 6009, Australia; demelza.ireland@uwa.edu.au
* Correspondence: zoya.gridneva@uwa.edu.au
† Presented at Australian Breastfeeding + Lactation Research and Science Translation Conference (ABREAST Conference 2024), Perth, Australia, 15 November 2024.

Keywords: multiple birth infants; twins; triplets; breastfeeding; lactation; breastfeeding characteristics; milk production; infant milk intake; barriers and facilitators

Breastfeeding multiple birth infants (MBIs) presents unique challenges that require tailored support and guidance, yet little research has focused on MBIs mothers experiences. This study employed a mixed methods approach and aimed to explore the breastfeeding journey of Australian mothers of MBIs, highlighting the barriers and facilitators they encounter and offering insights into breastfeeding experiences, maternal milk production, and infant milk intake. Data were collected between May and August 2024 via an online survey, which included both quantitative and qualitative components. Quantitative data focused on breastfeeding initiation, duration, and challenges, while qualitative data gathered the experiences, challenges, and support needs of mothers of MBIs. Thematic analysis was used to identify key themes from qualitative responses, and statistical analyses were performed to assess significant differences in breastfeeding outcomes between parity groups. A subset of participants participated in a 24 h milk profile study to measure maternal milk production and infant milk intake. Statistical significance was set at $p < 0.05$.

Survey data of $n = 151$ women ($n = 80$ primiparous, $n = 71$ multiparous) were available for analysis. This study revealed that, during pregnancy, 87.2% of mothers intended to breastfeed their MBIs. Commercial milk formula was typically introduced during the postnatal hospital stay, and 53.4% reported that they had achieved full breastfeeding during the first six months. The breastfeeding duration of those who had already ceased breastfeeding at the time of survey participation was 5 [3, 9] months. More than half of the infants in the survey were born preterm (58.3%), with NICU admission being the primary reason for the late initiation of breastfeeding. Overall, mothers of MBIs reported latching difficulties (56.0%), low milk supply (49.3%), and sore nipples (46.7%) as major barriers to breastfeeding. Among mothers with preterm infants, the significant barriers to breastfeeding included the need for supplementary feeds (80.2%), latching difficulties (54.9%), and infants' lack of energy (54.9%). The cost of lactation support did not hinder mothers' access to breastfeeding support and lactation aids, which likely reflects the higher socioeconomic status of the study sample. Nearly all mothers (98.7%) used electric breast pumps, which were followed by nursing pillows (89.2%) and nipple shields (44.6%) as the most commonly used lactation aids. The primary reason for expressing breast milk was to boost milk supply (68.2%) and to provide expressed breast milk (EBM) to other caregivers in order to feed infants (65.2%).

In the hospital, 71.6% of mothers reported satisfaction with breastfeeding support. However, qualitative data revealed the existence of a dichotomy in care experience, with some mothers receiving excellent hands-on support, while others reported feeling neglected due to busy staff or inconsistent advice. Many mothers reported that existing guidance and hospital support and education were primarily designed for mothers of singleton infants, leaving them unprepared to manage feeding of multiples. Mothers reported that improving breastfeeding outcomes requires specialized guidance, better access to lactation support, and in-home practical support to alleviate the burden of feeding and expressing. They also reported that healthcare professionals should be trained to offer practical, non-judgmental support, helping mothers to navigate the complex challenges of breastfeeding MBIs. This study underscores the need for MBI-specific breastfeeding education and consistent professional support, particularly in the early postpartum period, when establishing a robust milk supply is critical.

The analysis of the 24 h milk profiles in six mothers of twins showed that two mothers fed their twins directly from the breast for all feeds, one breastfed and supplemented with commercial milk formula, and three mothers exclusively expressed and fed both, EBM and commercial milk formula. On average, mothers produced 1403 ± 348 g of milk, with infants consuming on average 679 ± 206 g of mother's own milk with total infant milk intake being 813 ± 86 g, including commercial infant formula. While some mothers could produce sufficient milk volumes for their infants, maintaining milk supply required a significant time commitment. Mothers +/− other caregivers spent, on average, 5.0 ± 2.2 h feeding and expressing milk. This did not account for time spent cleaning feeding and expressing equipment, which further adds to the time-intensive demands required to feed MBIs.

This study illustrates the significant logistical, physical, and emotional challenges of breastfeeding MBIs. Providing early postpartum support, clinician training, and MBI-specific breastfeeding education and guidelines could help to improve breastfeeding outcomes as well as infant and maternal well-being.

Author Contributions: Conceptualization, M.A.G., Z.G. and D.T.G.; methodology, J.L.M., Z.G. and S.L.P.; formal analysis, M.A.G., Z.G. and S.L.P.; investigation, M.A.G.; resources, D.T.G.; data curation, J.L.M., A.H.W., Z.G. and S.L.P.; writing—original draft preparation, M.A.G.; writing—review and editing, J.L.M., A.H.W., D.J.I., D.T.G., Z.G. and S.L.P.; supervision, D.J.I., D.T.G., S.L.P. and Z.G.; project administration, J.L.M.; funding acquisition, D.T.G. All authors have read and agreed to the published version of the manuscript.

Funding: This research was funded by unrestricted research grant from Medela AG (Switzerland). The funder had no role in the design of the study; in the collection, analyses, or interpretation of data; in the writing of the manuscript; or in the decision to publish the results.

Institutional Review Board Statement: The study was conducted in accordance with the Declaration of Helsinki. The study was approved by the Human Research Ethics Committee at The University of Western Australia (2024/ET000324, RA/4/20/6134) and conducted in accordance with the relevant guidelines and regulations.

Informed Consent Statement: Informed consent was obtained from all subjects involved in the study.

Data Availability Statement: Restrictions apply to the availability of some, or all data generated or analyzed during this study. The corresponding author will on request detail the restrictions and any conditions under which access to some data may be provided.

Acknowledgments: We thank all of the participants for help with this research.

Conflicts of Interest: D.T.G. declares past participation in the Scientific Advisory Board of Medela AG. J.L.M., A.H.W., D.T.G., S.L.P. and Z.G. are supported by an unrestricted research grant from Medela AG, administered by The University of Western Australia. The funder had no role in the design of the study; in the collection, analyses, or interpretation of data; in the writing of the manuscript; or in the decision to publish the results. All other authors declare no conflicts of interest.

Disclaimer/Publisher's Note: The statements, opinions and data contained in all publications are solely those of the individual author(s) and contributor(s) and not of MDPI and/or the editor(s). MDPI and/or the editor(s) disclaim responsibility for any injury to people or property resulting from any ideas, methods, instructions or products referred to in the content.

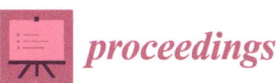

Abstract

Impact of Video-Based Breastfeeding Education on Self-Care Competencies of Postnatal Women [†]

Nalini Sirala Jagadeesh *, Sangavi Balaji and Rajeswari Singaravelu

Department of Obstetrics and Gynaecology Nursing, Sri Ramachandra Institute of Higher Education and Research (DU), Chennai 600 116, India; sangavi.b@sriramachandra.edu.in (S.B.); rajeswari.s@sriramachandra.edu.in (R.S.)
* Correspondence: sjnalini@sriramachandra.edu.in
[†] Presented at Australian Breastfeeding + Lactation Research and Science Translation Conference (ABREAST Conference 2024), Perth, Australia, 15 November 2024.

Keywords: breastfeeding; education; knowledge; skills; self-care competencies; postnatal women

Academic Editors: Donna T. Geddes and Zoya Gridneva

Published: 31 December 2024

Citation: Jagadeesh, N.S.; Balaji, S.; Singaravelu, R. Impact of Video-Based Breastfeeding Education on Self-Care Competencies of Postnatal Women. *Proceedings* 2025, 112, 2. https://doi.org/10.3390/proceedings2025112002

Copyright: © 2024 by the authors. Licensee MDPI, Basel, Switzerland. This article is an open access article distributed under the terms and conditions of the Creative Commons Attribution (CC BY) license (https://creativecommons.org/licenses/by/4.0/).

The postnatal period is a critical stage in the lives of both mothers and newborn infants [1]. Postnatal and newborn discharge education lacks standard teaching material, leading to unclear teaching at discharge and exposing unmet maternal expectations [2]. This study aimed to assess the effectiveness of video-based breastfeeding education in improving self-care competencies of postnatal women. The objectives of this study were to (a) examine the proportion of breastfeeding-related information received by women from healthcare providers before discharge and (b) develop and evaluate the effectiveness of a video-based breastfeeding education regarding self-care competencies of postnatal women. The study was conducted in two phases. In phase one, a survey, 130 postnatal women who were recruited through purposive sampling completed a 7-item five-point Likert scale questionnaire to express their satisfaction with breastfeeding information received before discharge from healthcare providers. The scale ranged from 5, fully satisfied, to 1, not satisfied. The overall scores were interpreted as <50%, inadequately satisfied; 50–75%, adequately satisfied; and >75%, highly satisfied. The postnatal women's satisfaction with addressing maternal questions or issues with breastfeeding by healthcare providers was also assessed (satisfied/dissatisfied). Based on these results, a video on breastfeeding education was prepared. In phase two, the impact of a video-based breastfeeding education program on postnatal women's self-care competencies was evaluated using a pre-experimental one-group pre-test post-test design. Self-care competencies included the knowledge and proficiency of postnatal women on breastfeeding and its technique. Fifty postnatal women completed a 12-item breastfeeding knowledge questionnaire before and after the intervention. The breastfeeding knowledge questionnaire had items related to breast milk characteristics, initiation of breastfeeding, exclusive breastfeeding, and breast care [3]. The breastfeeding knowledge questionnaire developed by the investigator was validated by nursing experts, and reliability was established using the test re-test method with a value of 0.7. Postnatal women's proficiency in breastfeeding their infants was observed before and after the intervention using the standardized LATCH tool [4] by research assistants who were blinded to postnatal women's exposure to video-based breastfeeding education. LATCH is a breastfeeding documentation tool that assigns a numerical score of 0, 1, or 2 to five key components of breastfeeding, such as latch, audible swallowing, type of nipple, comfort (breast/nipple), and hold (positioning), for a possible total score of

10 points. The key components were scored based on observation and interpreted as 0–3: poor, 4–7: moderate, and 8–10 as good. Frequency and percentages were used to assess the postnatal women's satisfaction with information received from healthcare providers before discharge and their satisfaction with information from healthcare providers' regarding the maternal questions/issues on breastfeeding. Mean and standard deviation are used to report the level of self-care competencies before and after intervention. A paired t-test was used to compare the differences in the self-care competencies before and after intervention. The results of phase one revealed that 11 (8.5%) postnatal women were highly satisfied and 96 (73.8%) were adequately satisfied with information received regarding breastfeeding before discharge. However, the majority of postnatal women (114 (87.6%)) expressed dissatisfaction with the healthcare providers' information on maternal questions/issues regarding breastfeeding. In phase two, the mean pre-test knowledge score on breastfeeding of 8.6 ±1.63 improved to 10.82 ± 1.77 ($p < 0.001$) in the post-test after the video-based breastfeeding education program. Observation showed that during the pre-test, 11 women (22%) had moderate LATCH scores and 39 women (78%) had good latching skills. Subsequently, in the post-test, 100% of postnatal women had good LATCH scores. This study concluded that women were not fully satisfied with the information from healthcare providers regarding maternal questions/issues on breastfeeding during discharge. Utilization of a well-developed, evidence-supported video-based breastfeeding education prior to discharge successfully enhanced the self-care competencies of postnatal women with breastfeeding.

Author Contributions: Conceptualization, N.S.J. and S.B.; Methodology, N.S.J. and S.B.; Validation, N.S.J., S.B. and R.S.; Formal analysis, S.B. and N.S.J.; Investigation, S.B.; Resources, N.S.J. and S.B.; Data curation S.B.; writing—original draft preparation, S.B. and N.S.J.; writing—review and editing, S.B., and R.S.; supervision, N.S.J. and R.S.; funding acquisition, S.B. All authors have read and agreed to the published version of the manuscript.

Funding: This research was self-funded by N.S.J.

Institutional Review Board Statement: The study was conducted in accordance with the Declaration of Helsinki and approved by the Institutional Ethics Committee for students in November 2022 (CSP/22/JUL/114/438).

Informed Consent Statement: Informed consent was obtained from all subjects involved in the study.

Data Availability Statement: Data sharing is not applicable.

Acknowledgments: We acknowledge the services of Urmila. U, Project Associate for statistical support, and the selected nurses for collecting post-test data in phase 2.

Conflicts of Interest: All the authors declare no conflicts of interest.

References

1. Ibrahim, M.A.; Mare, K.U.; Nur, M. Postnatal Care Utilization and Associated Factors among Mothers who gave Birth in the Aysaeta District, Northeast Ethiopia: A Community Based Cross-sectional Study. *Ethiop. J. Health Sci.* **2024**, *32*, 1123–1132. [CrossRef]
2. Dol, J.; Kohi, T.; Campbell-Yeo, M.; Murphy, G.T.; Aston, M.; Mselle, L. Exploring maternal postnatal newborn care postnatal discharge education in Dar es Salaam, Tanzania: Barriers, facilitators and opportunities. *Midwifery* **2019**, *77*, 137–143. [CrossRef] [PubMed]

6. Hamze, L.; Mao, J.; Reifsnider, E. Knowledge and attitudes towards breastfeeding practices: A cross-sectional survey of postnatal mothers in China. *Midwifery* **2019**, *74*, 68–75. [CrossRef]
7. Jensen, D.; Wallace, S.; Kelsay, P. LATCH: A Breastfeeding charting system and documentation Tool. *J. Obstet. Gynecol. Neonatal Nurs.* **1994**, *23*, 27–32. [CrossRef] [PubMed]

Disclaimer/Publisher's Note: The statements, opinions and data contained in all publications are solely those of the individual author(s) and contributor(s) and not of MDPI and/or the editor(s). MDPI and/or the editor(s) disclaim responsibility for any injury to people or property resulting from any ideas, methods, instructions or products referred to in the content.

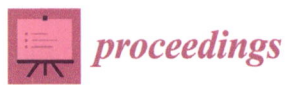

Abstract

Hormonal and Macronutrient Profiles in Human Milk Among Women with Low Milk Production [†]

Xuehua Jin [1,2,3], **Ching Tat Lai** [1,2,3], **Sharon L. Perrella** [1,2,3], **Jacki L. McEachran** [1,2,3], **Zoya Gridneva** [1,2,3] and **Donna T. Geddes** [1,2,3,*]

1. School of Molecular Sciences, The University of Western Australia, Crawley, WA 6009, Australia; xuehua.jin@research.uwa.edu.au (X.J.); ching-tat.lai@uwa.edu.au (C.T.L.); sharon.perrella@uwa.edu.au (S.L.P.); jacki.mceachran@uwa.edu.au (J.L.M.); zoya.gridneva@uwa.edu.au (Z.G.)
2. ABREAST Network, Perth, WA 6000, Australia
3. UWA Centre for Human Lactation Research and Translation, Crawley, WA 6009, Australia
* Correspondence: donna.geddes@uwa.edu.au
† Presented at Australian Breastfeeding + Lactation Research and Science Translation Conference (ABREAST Conference 2024), Perth, Australia, 15 November 2024.

Abstract: Adequate milk production is key for optimal infant growth, yet women often wean due to perceived low milk production (LMP). Maternal adiposity and gestational diabetes mellitus (GDM) are known potential risk factors for LMP and may alter both hormonal and macronutrient composition of human milk. This study aims to investigate the hormonal and macronutrient composition of human milk in relation to LMP particularly in the context of maternal adiposity and GDM. Human milk samples were collected from 68 women with LMP and 160 women with normal milk production during 1–6 months postpartum. Of the 228 participants with the mean pre-pregnancy BMI of 26.3 ± 6.0 kg/m^2, 80 (35.1%) had GDM. Concentrations of hormones (estrone, estradiol, progesterone, insulin, leptin, adiponectin) and macronutrients (fat, protein, lactose, glucose) were measured and compared between the two groups. Univariable and multivariable logistic regression analyses were conducted, adjusting for potential confounders such as maternal body mass index (BMI) and GDM, to assess the relationships between hormone and macronutrient concentrations, and milk production. Preliminary analyses indicated that higher concentrations of estrone ($p < 0.001$), leptin ($p = 0.009$), insulin ($p = 0.002$), protein ($p = 0.012$), and lactose ($p = 0.004$) were associated with LMP. After adjusting for maternal BMI and GDM in the univariable models, all of these associations remained, and progesterone ($p = 0.045$) also emerged as positively associated with LMP. In multivariable regression, followed by stepwise model selection, estrone ($p < 0.001$), protein ($p < 0.001$) and lactose ($p = 0.015$) demonstrated the strongest associations with LMP, with maternal BMI also contributing significantly ($p = 0.010$). The findings suggest that hormone and macronutrient concentrations in human milk may reflect LMP status and provide insights into the underlying biological mechanisms associated with LMP.

Keywords: human milk; breast milk; lactation; milk production; hormones; macronutrients; body mass index; gestational diabetes mellitus

Author Contributions: Conceptualization, X.J., C.T.L. and D.T.G.; methodology, C.T.L. and Z.G.; software, X.J. and C.T.L.; validation, X.J. and Z.G.; formal analysis, X.J.; investigation, X.J.; resources, D.T.G.; data curation, X.J., J.L.M. and Z.G.; writing—original draft preparation, X.J.; writing—review and editing, C.T.L., S.L.P., Z.G. and D.T.G.; visualization, X.J.; supervision, C.T.L., S.L.P. and D.T.G.; project administration, J.L.M.; funding acquisition, D.T.G. All authors have read and agreed to the published version of the manuscript.

Funding: C.T.L.: S.L.P., J.L.M., Z.G. and D.T.G. receive salaries from an unrestricted research grant from Medela AG (Switzerland) and administered by The University of Western Australia. X.J. is supported by UWA–China Scholarship Council (CSC) Joint PhD Scholarship and UWA–CSC Higher Degree by Research Top-Up Scholarship.

Institutional Review Board Statement: The study was conducted in accordance with the Declaration of Helsinki and was approved by The University of Western Australia Human Research Ethics Committee (2019/RA/4/20/6134).

Informed Consent Statement: Informed consent was obtained from all subjects involved in the study.

Data Availability Statement: Data sharing is not applicable.

Conflicts of Interest: D.T.G. declares participation in the Scientific Advisory Board of Medela AG. C.T.L., S.L.P., J.L.M., Z.G, and D.T.G. are/were supported by an unrestricted research grant from Medela AG, administered by UWA. The funders had no role in the design of the study; in the collection, analyses, or interpretation of data; in the writing of the manuscript; or in the decision to publish the results.

Disclaimer/Publisher's Note: The statements, opinions and data contained in all publications are solely those of the individual author(s) and contributor(s) and not of MDPI and/or the editor(s). MDPI and/or the editor(s) disclaim responsibility for any injury to people or property resulting from any ideas, methods, instructions or products referred to in the content.

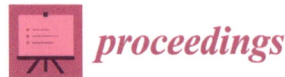 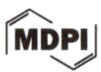

Abstract

Effect of Music Intervention on Breast Milk Volume and Stress Among Indian Preterm Mothers [†]

Rajeswari Singaravelu *, Temsurenla Jamir and Nalini Sirala Jagadeesh

Department of Obstetrics and Gynaecology Nursing, Sri Ramachandra Institute of Higher Education and Research (DU), Chennai 600116, India; temsurenjamir68@gmail.com (T.J.); sjnalini@sriramachandra.edu.in (N.S.J.)
* Correspondence: rajeswari.s@sriramachandra.edu.in
[†] Presented at Australian Breastfeeding + Lactation Research and Science Translation Conference (ABREAST Conference 2024), Perth, Australia, 15 November 2024.

Keywords: preterm infants; music; breast milk volume; stress; breast pump; breast milk expression

Nutrition is essential for preterm infants' growth, metabolism, and immunity [1–4]. The inadequate feeding capabilities of preterm infants and their higher nutritional requirements put pressure on mothers to produce and maintain an adequate milk supply, leading to maternal stress [5,6]. Music as a relaxation technique has been shown to reduce stress arousal and increase the quality and quantity of milk secretion, including its fat and calorie content [7–9]. Despite the proven benefits of music for stress reduction and milk secretion, it was of interest to study the effect of music intervention among breast pump-dependent preterm mothers. The objective was to assess the effect of music intervention on breast milk volume and stress among preterm mothers.

An open-label randomized controlled trial was conducted among 74 pump-dependent preterm mothers (37 each for the intervention and control groups) who delivered between 30 and 36 weeks of gestation and were admitted to a tertiary care university hospital in South India. All mothers were recruited on the third postnatal day and completed the post-test on the fifth postnatal day. Standardized Indian classical music (Hamsadhwani raga) was delivered through headphones for 30 min (15 min before and during the breast milk expression session) once a day for three consecutive days to the mothers in the intervention group. Breast milk volume was measured and recorded once a day for three days consistently between 10 and 11 am using a pocket weighing scale with the features of auto-calibration and tare full capacity. The calibration was manually tested daily using analytic weights. The weight (g) was converted to volume (mL) based on the density of human milk (1.03 g/mL). Stress was assessed using the Parental Stress Scale (PSS) by Berry and Jones [10] on the first and third day of intervention through interviews. Descriptive statistics were used to summarize participant characteristics, inferential statistics like independent t-tests were used to compare breast milk volume and stress scores between groups, and ANOVA was used to identify factors associated with these outcomes.

The results revealed that the mean gestational age was 32.95 ± 1.78 weeks in the intervention group and 32.96 ± 2.12 weeks in the control group. Other baseline characteristics were comparable between the groups. The average breast milk volume among the intervention group on the third day of intervention was 44.9 ± 7.48 mL, and for the control group, it was 33.17 ± 6.88 mL, with a mean difference of 11.73 mL (95% CI: 8.54–15.13, $p < 0.001$). The stress score among the intervention group was significantly lower (66.22 ± 3.30 vs. 68.97 ± 2.99 points) compared to the control group on the third day, with a mean difference of 2.73 points (95% CI: 1.53–3.87, $p < 0.001$). In the intervention group, maternal age

(18–23 years, $p = 0.007$), gestational age at birth (35–36 weeks, $p < 0.001$), the number of breast expression sessions per day (>8 sessions, $p = 0.004$), infant condition at birth (not intubated, $p = 0.009$), and the mode of thermoregulation (kangaroo mother care, $p = 0.001$) were significantly associated with expressed breast milk volume. Maternal body mass index (with obesity, $p = 0.028$) and the causes of preterm labor (premature rupture of membrane, $p = 0.043$) were the factors related to parental stress.

Music intervention is a cost-effective, non-invasive method that positively impacts stress reduction and is associated with an increase in breast milk volume among preterm mothers. This study highlights the potential benefits of targeted music intervention for breast pump-dependent preterm mothers for breast milk volume enhancement and stress reduction.

Author Contributions: Conceptualization, R.S. and T.J.; methodology, T.J.; validation, R.S., N.S.J. and T.J.; formal analysis, T.J. and R.S.; investigation, T.J.; resources, R.S. and T.J.; data curation, T.J.; writing—original draft preparation, T.J. and R.S.; writing—review and editing, T.J., R.S. and N.S.J.; supervision, R.S. and N.S.J.; funding acquisition, T.J. All authors have read and agreed to the published version of the manuscript.

Funding: This research was self-funded by R.S and T.J.

Institutional Review Board Statement: This study was conducted in accordance with the Declaration of Helsinki and approved by the Institutional Ethics Committee (CSP/18/APR/67/85, April 2018).

Informed Consent Statement: Informed consent was obtained from all subjects involved in the study.

Data Availability Statement: Data sharing is not applicable.

Acknowledgments: We thank U. Urmila for statistical support.

Conflicts of Interest: The authors declare no conflicts of interest.

References

1. Roggero, P.; Liotto, N.; Menis, C.; Mosca, F. New Insights in Preterm Nutrition. *Nutrients* **2020**, *12*, 1857. [CrossRef] [PubMed]
2. Diehl-Jones, W.L.; Askin, D.F. Nutritional Modulation of Neonatal Outcomes. *AACN Adv. Crit. Care* **2004**, *15*, 83–96. [CrossRef] [PubMed]
3. Stephens, B.E.; Vohr, B.R. Protein Intake and Neurodevelopmental Outcomes. *Clin. Perinatol.* **2014**, *41*, 323–329. [CrossRef] [PubMed]
4. Thoene, M.K.; Lyden, E.; Anderson-Berry, A. Improving nutrition outcomes for infants < 1500 grams with a progressive, evidenced-based enteral feeding protocol. *Nutr. Clin. Pract.* **2018**, *33*, 647–655. [CrossRef] [PubMed]
5. Abu Bakar, S.A.; Muda, S.M.; Arifin, S.R.M.; Ishak, S. Breast milk expression for premature infant in the neonatal intensive care unit: A review of mothers' perceptions. *Enferm. Clin.* **2019**, *29*, 725–732. [CrossRef]
6. Hill, P.D.; Aldag, J.C.; Chatterton, R.T.; Zinaman, M. Comparison of Milk Output Between Mothers of Preterm and Term Infants: The First 6 Weeks After Birth. *J. Hum. Lact.* **2005**, *21*, 22–30. [CrossRef] [PubMed]
7. Ak, J.; Lakshmanagowda, P.B.; Pradeep, G.C.M.; Goturu, J. Impact of music therapy on breast milk secretion in mothers of premature newborns. *J. Clin. Diagn. Res.* **2015**, *9*, CC04–CC06. [CrossRef] [PubMed]
8. SefidHaji, S.; Aziznejadroshan, P.; Mojaveri, M.H.; Nikbakht, H.A.; Qujeq, D.; Amiri, S.R.J. Effect of lullaby on volume, fat, total protein and albumin concentration of breast milk in premature infants' mothers admitted to NICU: A randomized controlled trial. *Int. Breastfeed. J.* **2022**, *17*, 71. [CrossRef] [PubMed]
9. Yu, J.; Wells, J.; Wei, Z.; Fewtrell, M. Effects of relaxation therapy on maternal psychological state, infant growth and gut microbiome: Protocol for a randomised controlled trial investigating mother-infant signalling during lactation following late preterm and early term delivery. *Int. Breastfeed. J.* **2019**, *14*, 50. [CrossRef] [PubMed]
10. Berry, J.O.; Jones, W.H. The Parental Stress Scale: Initial Psychometric Evidence. *J. Soc. Pers. Relatsh.* **1995**, *12*, 463–472. [CrossRef]

Disclaimer/Publisher's Note: The statements, opinions and data contained in all publications are solely those of the individual author(s) and contributor(s) and not of MDPI and/or the editor(s). MDPI and/or the editor(s) disclaim responsibility for any injury to people or property resulting from any ideas, methods, instructions or products referred to in the content.

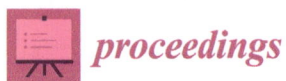

Abstract

Distinct Nutrient Sources and Infant Outcomes: Impact of Breastmilk and Complementary Food on Indonesian Infant Growth and Micronutrient Status [†]

Sofa Rahmannia [1,2,*], Kevin Murray [1], Gina Arena [3,4], Aly Diana [5] and Siobhan Hickling [1]

[1] School of Population and Global Health, The University of Western Australia, Nedlands, WA 6009, Australia
[2] Faculty of Medicine, Universitas Pasundan, Bandung 40117, Indonesia
[3] Medical School, The University of Western Australia, Perth, WA 6000, Australia
[4] Telethon Kids Institute, Nedlands, WA 6009, Australia
[5] Department of Public Health, Faculty of Medicine, Universitas Padjadjaran, Sumedang 45363, Indonesia
[*] Correspondence: sofa.rahmannia@research.uwa.edu.au
[†] Presented at Australian Breastfeeding + Lactation Research and Science Translation Conference (ABREAST Conference 2024), Perth, Australia, 15 November 2024.

Keywords: breastmilk composition; complementary feeding; infant growth; nutrient bioavailability; energy intake; zinc status; ferritin levels; longitudinal growth; infant nutrition

The relationship between infant nutrient intake and their nutritional status remains uncertain. Our previous study, which measured total intake from breastmilk (BM) and complementary food (CF), including infant formulas and cereal, found no significant association with growth and micronutrient status [1]. This study, conducted as part of an Indonesian breastfeeding cohort, aims to explore the relationship between intake from different sources, BM and CF, and nutritional outcomes, considering their differing nutrient profiles and bioavailability. Infant intake and growth were measured at 2 and 5 months of age, with iron (ferritin) and zinc (serum zinc) measured at 5 months. BM intake for energy was determined using creamatocrit analysis [2], while iron and zinc compositions were obtained by ICP-MS, then multiplied by individual milk volume measured by deuterium dose-to-mother [3]. CF intake was gathered by 3-day food records. Multivariable regression analysis was performed with intake as the predictor and growth and micronutrient biomarkers as the outcomes, adjusting for inflammation (CRP), breastfeeding practices (exclusive/partial), location (urban/rural), maternal age, and infant sex. Among 221 infants, mean anthropometric status at 5 months was low, with a height-for-age z-score (HAZ) of −0.8 (0.9), weight-for-age z-score (WAZ) of −0.6 (0.9), and weight-for-height z-score (WHZ) of 0.0 (1.0). The mean ferritin level was 35.9 ± 29.7 µg/L, and the mean zinc level was 10.4 ± 1.3 µmol/L. In partially breastfed infants, CF contributed 38% of total energy intake, 90% of iron intake, and 62% of zinc intake. Multivariable analysis revealed that only energy intake from BM was positively and significantly associated with infant growth, with every 100 kcal increase in BM energy associated with increases of 0.382 in HAZ ($p < 0.001$), 0.539 in WAZ ($p < 0.001$), and 0.383 in WHZ ($p < 0.001$). No correlation was observed between iron intake from either BM or CF with ferritin status at 5 months, but a positive correlation was found between zinc intake from BM and zinc status, with a 1.4 increase per mg of zinc intake ($p = 0.001$). No such correlation was observed with CF zinc intake and zinc status. These findings were consistent for intake at both 2 and 5 months in relation to growth, iron and zinc status. The lack of association between total infant diet and outcomes might be explained by differences in nutrient profiles from breastmilk and non-breastmilk sources

Analysing them separately could help clarify the association between dietary intake and infant outcomes. Monitoring BM composition as well as encouraging and supporting breastfeeding are crucial due to its potential to enhance infant nutrition.

Author Contributions: Conceptualization, S.R., S.H., G.A. and K.M.; methodology, S.R. and K.M.; formal analysis, S.R.; investigation, S.R. and A.D.; resources, A.D.; writing—original draft preparation, S.R.; writing—review and editing, S.H., G.A., K.M. and A.D.; supervision, S.H., G.A. and K.M.; project administration, S.R. and A.D. All authors have read and agreed to the published version of the manuscript.

Funding: This research was funded by Bill and Melinda Gates Foundation. The funder had no role in the design of the study; in the collection, analyses, or interpretation of data; in the writing of the manuscript; or in the decision to publish the results.

Institutional Review Board Statement: The study was conducted in accordance with the Declaration of Helsinki and approved by The University of Western Australia Human Research Ethic Committee (2022/ET000721) and by the Human Research Ethics Committee, Faculty of Medicine, Universitas Padjadjaran, Bandung, Indonesia (05/UN6.C1.3.2/KEPK/PN/2017).

Informed Consent Statement: Informed consent was obtained from all subjects involved in the study.

Data Availability Statement: The data supporting the conclusions of this article will be made available by the authors on request.

Acknowledgments: We would like to sincerely thank Rosalind Gibson and Lisa Houghton for their support during fieldwork, and Anna Alisjahbanna along with Frontiers for Health for their support in the community where data collection took place. We are also grateful to our research team—Dimas Erlangga Luftimas, Yenni Zuhairini, Annisha Fathonah, Wina Nur Sofiah, Aghnia Husnayiani Suryanto, Lina Sofiatul Inayah, Mohammad Brachim Anshari, and Afini Dwi Purnamasari—for their commitment and effort. Lastly, we extend our appreciation to the cadres and participants for their valuable involvement in this study.

Conflicts of Interest: The authors declare no conflicts of interest. The funders had no role in the design of the study; in the collection, analyses, or interpretation of data; in the writing of the manuscript; or in the decision to publish the results.

References

1. Leong, C.; Gibson, R.S.; Diana, A.; Haszard, J.J.; Rahmannia, S.; Ansari, M.B.; Inayah, L.S.; Purnamasari, A.D.; Houghton, L.A. Differences in micronutrient intakes of exclusive and partially breastfed Indonesian infants from resource-poor households are not accompanied by differences in micronutrient status, morbidity, or growth. *J. Nutr.* **2021**, *151*, 705–715. [CrossRef] [PubMed]
2. Meier, P.P.; Engstrom, J.L.; Zuleger, J.L.; Motykowski, J.E.; Vasan, U.; Meier, W.A.; Hartmann, P.E.; Williams, T.M. Accuracy of a user-friendly centrifuge for measuring creamatocrits on mothers' milk in the clinical setting. *Breastfeed. Med.* **2006**, *1*, 79–87. [CrossRef] [PubMed]
3. Liu, Z.; Diana, A.; Slater, C.; Preston, T.; Gibson, R.S.; Houghton, L.; Duffull, S.B. Development of a nonlinear hierarchical model to describe the disposition of deuterium in mother-infant pairs to assess exclusive breastfeeding practice. *J. Pharmacokinet. Pharmacodyn.* **2019**, *46*, 1–13. [CrossRef] [PubMed]

Disclaimer/Publisher's Note: The statements, opinions and data contained in all publications are solely those of the individual author(s) and contributor(s) and not of MDPI and/or the editor(s). MDPI and/or the editor(s) disclaim responsibility for any injury to people or property resulting from any ideas, methods, instructions or products referred to in the content.

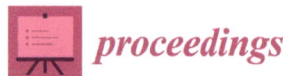 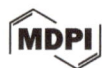

Abstract

Maternal Factors That Influence the Presence of Food Allergens in Human Milk—A Systematic Review [†]

Sophie A. Hughes [1,2,3,4], Zoya Gridneva [1,2,3], Sharon L. Perrella [1,2,3], Donna T. Geddes [1,2,3] and Debra J. Palmer [4,5,*]

[1] School of Molecular Sciences, The University of Western Australia, Crawley, WA 6009, Australia; sophie.hughes@research.uwa.edu.au (S.A.H.); zoya.gridneva@uwa.edu.au (Z.G.); sharon.perrella@uwa.edu.au (S.L.P.); donna.geddes@uwa.edu.au (D.T.G.)
[2] ABREAST Network, Perth, WA 6000, Australia
[3] UWA Centre for Human Lactation Research and Translation, Crawley, WA 6009, Australia
[4] The Kids Research Institute Australia, The University of Western Australia, Nedlands, WA 6009, Australia
[5] School of Medicine, The University of Western Australia, Crawley, WA 6009, Australia
* Correspondence: debbie.palmer@uwa.edu.au
[†] Presented at Australian Breastfeeding + Lactation Research and Science Translation Conference (ABREAST Conference 2024), Perth, Australia, 15 November 2024.

Abstract: Food allergens have been detected in human milk with wide frequency and concentration variations between women. As maternal factors such as age, body mass index (BMI), and allergic disease influence human milk composition, we aimed to identify which maternal characteristics have previously been associated with the presence of food allergens in milk. We conducted a systematic review search in MEDLINE, EMBASE, Cochrane Library, CINAHL, and Scopus, with inclusion criteria of common food allergens, human studies published in English with 10 or more participants providing milk samples, trials, observational studies, letters to the editor, and short communications. We obtained 5125 articles and 4127 after duplicates were removed. After the initial screening, 51 articles underwent full-text assessment, with a final 31 articles included in the analysis. A systematic review tool was used to extract all article information. We found that when a standardized amount of food allergen was consumed (16/31 studies), there were large inter-women variations in the frequency and concentrations of food allergens detected in human milk. The most common maternal characteristics that were investigated to determine their potential to influence the presence of food allergens in human milk were maternal allergic disease, usual diet, and weeks of lactation. Two studies found that if a woman's diet contained a specific food allergen, this influenced the detection of that food allergen in milk, while three studies found no such influence. Maternal allergic disease positively influenced the detection of food allergens in 3 studies, while 10 studies found no significant associations. Although data on other maternal characteristics, such as BMI, ethnicity, smoking, and parity, were recorded in some studies, these were not investigated for their influence on the presence of food allergens in human milk. Hence, although many studies reported maternal characteristics, most did not explore their associations with food allergens detected in milk. Future research investigating maternal characteristics that influence the presence of food allergens in human milk is needed to contribute to targeted food allergy prevention strategies.

Keywords: food allergies; food proteins; human milk; maternal factors

Academic Editors: Nicolas L. Taylor and Ching Tat Lai

Published: 2 January 2025

Citation: Hughes, S.A.; Gridneva, Z.; Perrella, S.L.; Geddes, D.T.; Palmer, D.J. Maternal Factors That Influence the Presence of Food Allergens in Human Milk—A Systematic Review. *Proceedings* **2025**, *112*, 6. https://doi.org/10.3390/proceedings2025112006

Copyright: © 2025 by the authors. Licensee MDPI, Basel, Switzerland. This article is an open access article distributed under the terms and conditions of the Creative Commons Attribution (CC BY) license (https://creativecommons.org/licenses/by/4.0/).

Author Contributions: Conceptualization S.A.H., S.L.P., D.T.G. and D.J.P.; methodology, D.J.P. and Z.G.; investigation, S.A.H. and D.J.P.; data curation, S.A.H., D.J.P. and Z.G.; writing—original draft preparation, S.A.H.; writing—review and editing, Z.G., S.L.P., D.T.G. and D.J.P.; supervision, S.L.P., D.T.G., D.J.P. and Z.G. All authors have read and agreed to the published version of the manuscript.

Funding: S.A.H. is supported by an Australian Government Research Training Program Domestic Fees Offset Scholarship and an Australian Government Research Training Stipend. Z.G., S.L.P., and D.T.G. are supported by an unrestricted research grant from Medela AG (Switzerland), administered by The University of Western Australia. D.J.P. is supported by The Kids Research Institute Australia Ascend Fellowship.

Institutional Review Board Statement: Systematic review was registered with PROSPERO (CRD42024558231).

Informed Consent Statement: Not applicable.

Data Availability Statement: Not applicable.

Conflicts of Interest: D.T.G. declares participation in the Scientific Advisory Board of Medela AG. D.T.G., S.L.P., and Z.G. receive funding from Medela AG, administered by The University of Western Australia. The funders had no role in the design of the study, in the collection, analysis, or interpretation of data, in the writing of the manuscript, or in the decision to publish the results.

Disclaimer/Publisher's Note: The statements, opinions and data contained in all publications are solely those of the individual author(s) and contributor(s) and not of MDPI and/or the editor(s). MDPI and/or the editor(s) disclaim responsibility for any injury to people or property resulting from any ideas, methods, instructions or products referred to in the content.

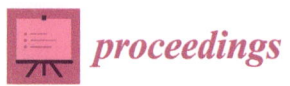

Abstract

Efficacy Assessment of the Breast Shield Size [†]

Zoya Gridneva [1,2,3,*], Ashleigh H. Warden [1,2,3], Jacki L. McEachran [1,2,3], Sharon L. Perrella [1,2,3], Ching Tat Lai [1,2,3] and Donna T. Geddes [1,2,3]

1. School of Molecular Sciences, The University of Western Australia, Crawley, WA 6009, Australia; ashleigh.warden@uwa.edu.au (A.H.W.); jacki.mceachran@uwa.edu.au (J.L.M.); sharon.perrella@uwa.edu.au (S.L.P.); ching-tat.lai@uwa.edu.au (C.T.L.); donna.geddes@uwa.edu.au (D.T.G.)
2. ABREAST Network, Perth, WA 6000, Australia
3. UWA Centre for Human Lactation Research and Translation, Crawley, WA 6009, Australia
* Correspondence: zoya.gridneva@uwa.edu.au; Tel.: +61-8-6488-4467
† Presented at Australian Breastfeeding + Lactation Research and Science Translation Conference (ABREAST Conference 2024), Perth, Australia, 15 November 2024.

Keywords: lactation; breastfeeding; human milk; breast pumping; breast expression; electric breast pump; nipple shield size; nipple diameter and length

Academic Editors: Nicolas L. Taylor and Debbie Palmer

Published: 2 January 2025

Citation: Gridneva, Z.; Warden, A.H.; McEachran, J.L.; Perrella, S.L.; Lai, C.T.; Geddes, D.T.. Efficacy Assessment of the Breast Shield Size. *Proceedings* **2025**, *112*, 7. https://doi.org/10.3390/proceedings2025112007

Copyright: © 2025 by the authors. Licensee MDPI, Basel, Switzerland. This article is an open access article distributed under the terms and conditions of the Creative Commons Attribution (CC BY) license (https://creativecommons.org/licenses/by/4.0/).

The diameters of the milk ducts increase significantly (2.5 ± 1.5 mm) with milk ejection as oxytocin is released, and then decrease, as oxytocin decreases, during a breastfeeding session [1]. As the main milk ducts, beneath the areola, are located superficially, they have the potential to be compressed by the breast shield during pumping. To overcome the most common concerns with pumping (a low volume and/or discomfort), there has been a focus on the correct fitting of the breast shields. Recommendations range from fitting the breast shield to nipple dimensions to allowing a 4 mm gap to allow the smooth movement of the breast and nipple without the undue compression of either.

Given discrepancies in recommendations, we investigated breast shield fitting with respect to pumping efficacy, maternal perception, and comfort. Lactating mothers (n = 157, 212 sessions) participated in one to three standard pumping sessions (two sessions, n = 52; three sessions n = 1) where either the same or a different breast (n = 4) was pumped, and nipple measurements were made prior to pumping. At the pumping session, with an electric breast pump that applies a Medela 2-phase expression pattern (M2-PEP, Medela AG, Baar, Switzerland), the stimulation pattern was applied for 2 min or until the first milk flow/ejection, after which the pattern was switched to the expression mode and pumping continued for 15 min. Mothers completed a 24 h milk production (24 h MP) profile to allow the degree of fullness (DOF) of the breast pre- and post-expression and the percentage of available milk removed (PAMR) to be calculated. We compared comfort and milk removal parameters during pumping sessions of a group in which the breast shield was fitted appropriately, with a 21 mm or larger shield (FA21>; n = 89, 105 sessions), to three other groups: one in which the breast shield was not fitted appropriately (or could not be fitted) for various, including physiological, reasons (NFA; all sizes, n = 87, 107 sessions); a group that could be fitted with a shield of 18 mm or smaller (NFA18<; n = 55, 71 sessions); and a group in which a smaller-than-appropriately fitted shield was used, i.e., with <4 mm space (NFAS; n = 10, 12 sessions). For statistical analysis, we used unpaired t-tests and linear mixed effect models accounting for DOF pre-expression and/or maximum comfortable vacuum applied and participant as a random effect.

During the first pumping session, 62% (98/157) of mothers were fitted with a 21 mm shield, 35% (55/157) with a 24 mm shield, and 3% (4/157) with a shield size of 27 mm. The protocol (4 mm) was to use the same shield size at consecutive sessions, unless a change was requested by the participant. Out of 49 mothers that attended multiple sessions and pumped the same breast, based on their nipple measurements, 17 mothers (35%) could be fitted differently (a smaller or larger shield size) at the consecutive session, including with a <21 mm shield ($n = 5$, 10%). Three participants (6%) were fitted with a different shield size at the consecutive session.

The comfort levels at the start and the end of milk expression were similar between FA21> and the other groups. The maximum comfortable vacuum was weaker in the NFAS group compared to FA21> (-181 ± 43 vs. -211 ± 51 mmHg, respectively; $p = 0.047$).

No significant difference was observed between the groups for the volume of milk removed, DOF, PAMR, or milk removal efficacy ratio (g/min). In multivariable models, the milk volume removed and PAMR, as well as the DOF post-expression, did not differ by the shield size or by the extent of the shield being oversized. Further, the volume of milk removed and PAMR were not associated with the nipple diameters, length, or temperature pre- or post-expression or with changes in these parameters pre-/post-expression.

This study found that despite the unintended doubling (8 mm on average) of the recommended breast shield tunnel width, this resulted in no difference in breast emptying efficacy or comfort during pumping. Whilst the correct fitting of the breast shield is essential for successful pumping, pumping with a bigger shield may not necessarily be detrimental to pumping performance or comfort. Further investigations are needed into pumping with directly fitted or smaller shields.

Author Contributions: Conceptualization, Z.G. and D.T.G.; methodology, A.H.W., J.L.M., C.T.L., S.L.P. and Z.G.; data collection, Z.G., and A.H.W.; formal analysis, Z.G.; investigation, Z.G. and A.H.W.; resources, D.T.G.; data curation, Z.G., A.H.W., J.L.M. and S.L.P.; writing—original draft preparation, Z.G.; writing—review and editing, A.H.W., J.L.M., S.L.P, C.T.L. and D.T.G.; supervision, D.T.G.; project administration, J.L.M.; funding acquisition, D.T.G. All authors have read and agreed to the published version of the manuscript.

Funding: This research was funded by an unrestricted research grant from Medela AG (Switzerland). The funder had no role in the design of the study; in the collection, analyses, or interpretation of data; in the writing of the manuscript; or in the decision to publish the results.

Institutional Review Board Statement: This study was conducted in accordance with the Declaration of Helsinki. The study was approved by the Human Research Ethics Committee at The University of Western Australia (RA/4/20/6407) and conducted in accordance with the relevant guidelines and regulations.

Informed Consent Statement: Informed consent was obtained from all subjects involved in the study.

Data Availability Statement: Restrictions apply to the availability of some or all data generated or analyzed during this study. The corresponding author will, on request, detail the restrictions and any conditions under which access to some data may be provided.

Acknowledgments: We thank all of the participants for their help with breastfeeding research.

Conflicts of Interest: D.T.G. declares past participation in the Scientific Advisory Board of Medela AG. All authors are/were supported by an unrestricted research grant from Medela AG, administered by The University of Western Australia. The funders had no role in the design of the study; in the collection, analyses, or interpretation of data; in the writing of the manuscript; or in the decision to publish the results. All other authors declare no conflicts of interest.

Reference

1. Ramsay, D.T.; Kent, J.C.; Owens, R.A.; Hartmann, P.E. Ultrasound imaging of milk ejection in the breast of lactating women. *Pediatrics* **2004**, *113*, 361–367. [CrossRef]

Disclaimer/Publisher's Note: The statements, opinions and data contained in all publications are solely those of the individual author(s) and contributor(s) and not of MDPI and/or the editor(s). MDPI and/or the editor(s) disclaim responsibility for any injury to people or property resulting from any ideas, methods, instructions or products referred to in the content.

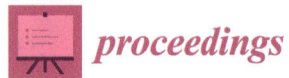

Abstract

Breastfeeding Longitudinal Observational Study of Mothers and Kids—BLOSOM Cohort †

Zoya Gridneva [1,2,3,*], Ali S. Cheema [4], Erika M. van den Dries [1], Ashleigh H. Warden [1,2,3], Jacki L. McEachran [1,2,3], Sharon L. Perrella [1,2,3], Ching Tat Lai [1,2,3], Lisa F. Stinson [1,2,3] and Donna T. Geddes [1,2,3]

1. School of Molecular Sciences, The University of Western Australia, Perth, WA 6009, Australia; vandendries@iinet.net.au (E.M.v.d.D.); ashleigh.warden@uwa.edu.au (A.H.W.); jacki.mceachran@uwa.edu.au (J.L.M.); sharon.perrella@uwa.edu.au (S.L.P.); ching-tat.lai@uwa.edu.au (C.T.L.); lisa.stinson@uwa.edu.au (L.F.S.); donna.geddes@uwa.edu.au (D.T.G.)
2. ABREAST Network, Perth, WA 6000, Australia
3. UWA Centre for Human Lactation Research and Translation, Perth, WA 6009, Australia
4. The Kids Research Institute Australia, Perth, WA 6009, Australia; alisadiq.cheema@telethonkids.org.au
* Correspondence: zoya.gridneva@uwa.edu.au; Tel.: +61-8-6488-4467
† Presented at Australian Breastfeeding + Lactation Research and Science Translation Conference (ABREAST Conference 2024), Perth, Australia, 15 November 2024.

Keywords: lactation; breastfeeding; human milk; infants; mothers; microbiome; human milk composition; body composition; growth; intake

The Breastfeeding Longitudinal Observational Study of Mothers and kids (BLOSOM) is a single-centre prospective cohort study conducted in Perth (Western Australia) that collected data from 2018 to 2020 and aimed to investigate the mechanisms by which human milk affects infant growth, health, and body composition. Pregnant women ($n = 119$) were recruited from the community and online networks during the third trimester of pregnancy (>30 weeks gestation). Inclusion criteria were women self-reported as healthy with no major pregnancy complications, intention to exclusively breastfeed up to at least 5 months postpartum, and intention to breastfeed until 12 months postpartum. Exclusion criteria included maternal smoking and pregnancy complications, such as preterm labour, preeclampsia, and gestational diabetes mellitus. All participants provided informed written consent to participate in the study, which was approved by the Human Research Ethics Committee at The University of Western Australia (RA/4/20/4023). Twenty-two participants withdrew from the study for various reasons, with $n = 97$ dyads remaining in the study (97 mothers and 99 infants). Mothers provided a milk sample and answered a demographic background questionnaire at the time of recruitment and an infant and maternal questionnaire during the sample collection day at the follow-up visits (days 2–5, and then months 1, 2, 3, 4, 5, 6, 9, 12, and 24). The samples collected were maternal and infant faeces, human milk, and infant oral swabs. The 24 h milk profile including maternal 24 h milk production and 24 h infant intake of human milk was measured at 3, 9, and 12 months postpartum. Maternal and infant anthropometrics as well as body composition using a bioelectrical impedance analyser ImpediMed SFB7 (ImpediMed, Brisbane, Queensland, Australia) were measured at 3, 6, 9, 12, and 24 months postpartum. Infant and maternal questionnaires collected information on maternal diet and maternal and infant health, including previous medical or surgical history and allergies, current medication including antibiotics, current smoking, the use of commercial milk formula and solid foods, dummy use, the use of a breast pump and nipple shield, nipple pain and trauma, childcare attendance, and pets in home. The cohort description was previously briefly included in several papers that reported major findings in this population [1–6].

Author Contributions: Conceptualization, A.S.C. and D.T.G.; methodology, E.M.v.d.D., D.T.G., C.T.L., L.F.S. and Z.G.; data collection, A.S.C. and E.M.v.d.D.; formal analysis, A.S.C., C.T.L., A.H.W., L.F.S. and Z.G; investigation, A.S.C., E.M.v.d.D., C.T.L., A.H.W, L.F.S., Z.G. and D.T.G.; resources, D.T.G.; data curation, Z.G., A.H.W., A.S.C., E.M.v.d.D., J.L.M., L.F.S. and S.L.P.; writing—original draft preparation, Z.G.; writing—review and editing, A.S.C., E.M.v.d.D., A.H.W., J.L.M., S.L.P., C.T.L., L.F.S. and D.T.G.; supervision, D.T.G.; project administration, J.L.M.; funding acquisition, D.T.G. All authors have read and agreed to the published version of the manuscript.

Funding: This research was funded by an unrestricted research grant from Medela AG (Switzerland) administered by The University of Western Australia. A.S.C. was supported by an additional SIRF (Scholarships for International Research Fees) scholarship from The University of Western Australia. The funders had no role in the design of the study; in the collection, analyses, or interpretation of data; in the writing of the manuscript; or in the decision to publish the results.

Institutional Review Board Statement: The study was conducted in accordance with the Declaration of Helsinki. The study was approved by the Human Research Ethics Committee at The University of Western Australia (RA/4/20/4023) and conducted in accordance with the relevant guidelines and regulations.

Informed Consent Statement: Informed consent was obtained from all subjects involved in the study.

Data Availability Statement: Restrictions apply to the availability of some or all data generated or analysed during this study. The corresponding author will detail on request the restrictions and any conditions under which access to some data may be provided.

Acknowledgments: We thank all of the participants for help with the breastfeeding research.

Conflicts of Interest: D.T.G. declares past participation in the Scientific Advisory Board of Medela AG. Z.G., A.S.C., E.M.D., A.H.W., J.L.M., S.L.P., C.T.L., L.F.S. and D.T.G are/were supported by an unrestricted research grant from Medela AG, administered by The University of Western Australia. A.S.C. was supported by an additional SIRF (Scholarships for International Research Fees) scholarship from The University of Western Australia. The funders had no role in the design of the study; in the collection, analyses, or interpretation of data; in the writing of the manuscript; or in the decision to publish the results.

References

1. Cheema, A.S.; Stinson, L.F.; Rea, A.; Lai, C.T.; Payne, M.S.; Murray, K.; Geddes, D.T.; Gridneva, Z. Human milk lactose, insulin, and glucose relative to infant body composition during exclusive breastfeeding. *Nutrients* **2021**, *13*, 3724. [CrossRef]
2. Bilston-John, S.H.; Narayanan, A.; Lai, C.T.; Rea, A.; Joseph, J.; Geddes, D.T. Macro- and trace-element intake from human milk in Australian infants: Inadequacy with respect to national recommendations. *Nutrients* **2021**, *13*, 3548. [CrossRef] [PubMed]
3. Cheema, A.S.; Gridneva, Z.; Furst, A.J.; Roman, A.S.; Trevenen, M.L.; Turlach, B.A.; Lai, C.T.; Stinson, L.F.; Bode, L.; Payne, M.S.; et al. Human milk oligosaccharides and bacterial profile modulate infant body composition during exclusive breastfeeding. *Int. J. Mol. Sci.* **2022**, *23*, 2865. [CrossRef]
4. Cheema, A.S.; Trevenen, M.L.; Turlach, B.A.; Furst, A.J.; Roman, A.S.; Bode, L.; Gridneva, Z.; Lai, C.T.; Stinson, L.F.; Payne, M.S.; et al. Exclusively breastfed infant microbiota develops over time and is associated with human milk oligosaccharide intakes. *Int. J. Mol. Sci.* **2022**, *23*, 2804. [CrossRef] [PubMed]

5. Suwaydi, M.A.; Lai, C.T.; Rea, A.; Gridneva, Z.; Perrella, S.L.; Wlodek, M.E.; Geddes, D.T. Circadian Variation in Human Milk Hormones and Macronutrients. *Nutrients* **2023**, *15*, 3729. [CrossRef] [PubMed]
6. Suwaydi, M.A.; Lai, C.T.; Warden, A.H.; Perrella, S.L.; McEachran, J.L.; Wlodek, M.E.; Geddes, D.T.; Gridneva, Z. Investigation of relationships between intakes of human milk total lipids and metabolic hormones and infant sex and body composition. *Nutrients* **2024**, *16*, 2739. [CrossRef] [PubMed]

Disclaimer/Publisher's Note: The statements, opinions and data contained in all publications are solely those of the individual author(s) and contributor(s) and not of MDPI and/or the editor(s). MDPI and/or the editor(s) disclaim responsibility for any injury to people or property resulting from any ideas, methods, instructions or products referred to in the content.

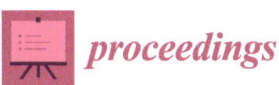

Abstract

Milk Ejections and Milk Flow Patterns During Breast Expression: When to Stop Pumping [†]

Zoya Gridneva [1,2,3,*], **Ashleigh H. Warden** [1,2,3], **Jacki L. McEachran** [1,2,3], **Sharon L. Perrella** [1,2,3], **Ching Tat Lai** [1,2,3] **and Donna T. Geddes** [1,2,3]

1. School of Molecular Sciences, The University of Western Australia, Crawley, WA 6009, Australia; ashleigh.warden@uwa.edu.au (A.H.W.); jacki.mceachran@uwa.edu.au (J.L.M.); sharon.perrella@uwa.edu.au (S.L.P.); ching-tat.lai@uwa.edu.au (C.T.L.); donna.geddes@uwa.edu.au (D.T.G.)
2. ABREAST Network, Perth, WA 6000, Australia
3. UWA Centre for Human Lactation Research and Translation, Crawley, WA 6009, Australia
* Correspondence: zoya.gridneva@uwa.edu.au; Tel.: +61-8-6488-4467
† Presented at Australian Breastfeeding + Lactation Research and Science Translation Conference (ABREAST Conference 2024), Perth, Australia, 15 November 2024.

Keywords: lactation; breastfeeding; human milk; breast pumping; breast expression; electric breast pump; pumping time; degree of fullness of the breast; milk ejection; milk removal

Despite the available evidence, mothers often do not tailor the duration of their pumping sessions to their individual milk flow pattern. Therefore, many mothers miss the opportunity to save time whilst effectively pumping their milk and maintaining their milk supply. This is particularly important for mothers that are pump-dependent, such as after preterm birth, when they need to pump 6–8 times per day. Milk ejection (ME) patterns are consistent within mothers, so while most mothers have several MEs earlier in the pumping session, others may have continuous milk flow [1]. However, milk flow patterns and the time of active milk removal during a pumping session have not been extensively characterized. We aimed to describe MEs, milk flow and milk removal patterns as well as the efficacy of milk removal and comfort during a standard Symphony (Medela AG, Baar, Switzerland) session. We also described the effects of breast fullness and late MEs on milk removal parameters.

Lactating mothers 3.8 ± 1.4 months postpartum ($n = 147$) participated in one to three standard Symphony sessions ($n = 225$) using a standard fitted shield and maximum comfortable vacuum (MCV). Mothers completed a 24 h milk production profile to allow for the calculation of the pre- and post-expression degree of fullness of the breast (DOF) and the percentage of available milk removed (PAMR). We used a continuous weighing balance to determine changes in milk flow rate [2]. The two predominant milk flow patterns during pumping were as follows: a few defined MEs (Pattern 1, ≤ 4 MEs) and many defined MEs (Pattern 2, ≥ 5 MEs). Sessions with late MEs (MEs that occurred ≥ 3 min after milk flow stopped) were also investigated. Linear mixed effect models were used to evaluate the effects of milk flow patterns on the efficacy of milk removal and other relationships between milk removal parameters. When two Symphony sessions ($n = 76$) were completed by the same participant, DOF pre-expression was categorized as 'emptier' or 'fuller', and paired t-tests were conducted to compare the two sessions. Mothers completed a single pumping session ($n = 71$), two sessions ($n = 74$) or three sessions ($n = 2$). Overall, the average amount of milk removed, PAMR and number of MEs was 76 ± 49 g, $66 \pm 26\%$ and 4.5 ± 1.6, respectively. Milk flow patterns were consistent within mothers, and the two patterns were equally represented between mothers: Pattern 1: single sessions (55%), double (51%); Pattern 2: single sessions (45%), double (27%).

Degree of fullness: A higher pre-expression DOF was observed with Pattern 2 (0.49 (0.14), $p < 0.001$) and a higher number of MEs (1.34 (0.41), $p = 0.002$). More milk was removed with Pattern 2 (12.02 (5.66) g, $p = 0.038$) with a higher number of MEs (4.59 (1.91) g, $p = 0.020$). If the breast was fuller when pumped, creamatocrit post-expression (fuller: 13.7 ± 4.8%; emptier: 12.6 ± 4.2%; $p = 0.037$), DOF pre-expression (fuller: 0.82 ± 0.18; emptier: 0.62 ± 0.23; $p < 0.001$) and the volume of milk removed (fuller: 91 ± 54 g; emptier: 67 ± 44 g; $p < 0.001$) were higher. The efficacy ratios of milk removal were higher when the fuller breast was pumped: milk removal rate (fuller: 6.1 ± 3.6 g/min; emptier: 4.3 ± 2.9 g/min; $p < 0.001$), constant flow rate (fuller: 9.3 ± 4.7 g/min; emptier: 8.2 ± 4.5 g/min; $p = 0.009$), milk removed during constant flow (fuller: 79 ± 54 g; emptier: 57 ± 42 g; $p < 0.001$) and active milk removal (fuller: 8.4 ± 5.0 g/min; emptier: 6.8 ± 4.0 g/min; $p < 0.001$). The time when pumping could stop did not differ by the fullness of the breast (fuller: 11.6 ± 3.3 min; emptier: 11.7 ± 3.6 min; $p = 0.45$); however, when the fuller breast was pumped, more milk was expressed at time to stop (fuller: 85 ± 51 g; emptier: 64 ± 42 g; $p < 0.001$) with a higher efficacy ratio (fuller: 7.8 ± 4.9 g/min; emptier: 6.1 ± 4.4 g/min; $p < 0.001$).

Milk flow: Longer active flow durations (AFDs) and constant flow durations (CFDs) and higher efficacy ratios were associated with a higher PAMR (AFD: 1.83 (0.55)%, $p = 0.002$; CFD: 1.93 (0.56)%, $p = 0.001$) and a larger volume of milk removed (AFD: 3.22 (0.83) g, $p < 0.001$; CFD: 4.57 (0.68) g, $p < 0.001$). Milk volume removed at a late ME was positively associated with the total volume of milk removed (1.73 (0.60) g, $p = 0.035$). The maximum flow rate was higher (fuller: 0.47 ± 0.27 g/s; emptier: 0.43 ± 0.25 g/s; $p = 0.012$), and both AFDs (fuller: 11.2 ± 3.4 min; emptier: 10.3 ± 3.3 min; $p = 0.005$) and CFDs (fuller: 8.8 ± 4.2 min; emptier: 7.2 ± 3.6 min; $p < 0.001$) were longer when the fuller breast was pumped. However, overall and non-flow durations were not significantly different. Milk flow patterns did not differ significantly between sessions, but a higher number of MEs was observed when the fuller breast was pumped (fuller: 4.7 ± 1.6; emptier: 4.4 ± 1.5; $p = 0.015$). The time to the first milk flow (fuller: 0.69 ± 0.74 min; emptier: 1.04 ± 1.54 min; $p = 0.035$) and to the first ME (fuller: 1.12 ± 0.82 min; emptier: 1.66 ± 2.14 min; $p = 0.028$) were shorter.

Nipple temperature: Higher post-expression nipple temperatures (°C) were associated with Pattern 2 (0.06 (0.03), $p = 0.037$) and a higher number of MEs (0.25 (0.08), $p = 0.003$), as well as increased flow durations (overall flow duration: 0.11 (0.03) °C, $p = 0.001$; AFD: 0.07 (0.03) °C, $p = 0.021$; CFD: 0.06 (0.03) °C, $p = 0.047$; time to stop pumping: 0.08 (0.03) °C, $p = 0.006$; time to last ME: 0.11 (0.02) °C, $p < 0.001$; and time to late ME: 0.20 (0.07) °C, $p = 0.037$). Higher post-expression nipple temperatures were also related to higher amounts of milk expressed (total milk removed: 0.005 (0.002) °C, $p = 0.027$; milk removed during CFD: 0.006 (0.003) °C, $p = 0.016$; milk at time to stop pumping: 0.006 (0.003) °C, $p = 0.031$; milk after time to stop: 0.09 (0.04) °C, $p = 0.017$ and higher efficacy ratio (milk removal rate, g/min): 0.08 (0.04) °C, $p = 0.036$).

Our findings show that the pre-expression degree of fullness of the breast drives most of the relationships with milk flow patterns and efficacy parameters. Further, pumping a fuller breast results in more milk removed and higher efficacy ratios; however, the overall flow duration time and PAMR are not affected, indicating that for individual women, breast drainage occurs at the same time regardless of the degree of breast fullness. Therefore, most mothers can pump for less than 15 min independent of the fullness of the breast to remove most of the available milk.

Author Contributions: Conceptualization, Z.G. and D.T.G.; methodology, A.H.W., J.L.M., C.T.L., S.L.P. and Z.G.; data collection, Z.G. and A.H.W.; formal analysis, Z.G.; investigation, Z.G. and A.H.W.; resources, D.T.G.; data curation, Z.G., A.H.W., J.L.M. and S.L.P.; writing—original draft preparation, Z.G.; writing—review and editing, A.H.W., J.L.M., S.L.P., C.T.L. and D.T.G.; supervision, D.T.G.; project administration, J.L.M.; funding acquisition, D.T.G. All authors have read and agreed to the published version of the manuscript.

Funding: This research was funded by an unrestricted research grant from Medela AG (Switzerland). The funder had no role in the design of the study; in the collection, analyses or interpretation of data; in the writing of the manuscript or in the decision to publish the results.

Institutional Review Board Statement: This study was conducted in accordance with the Declaration of Helsinki. This study was approved by the Human Research Ethics Committee at The University of Western Australia (RA/4/20/6407) and conducted in accordance with the relevant guidelines and regulations.

Informed Consent Statement: Informed consent was obtained from all subjects involved in this study.

Data Availability Statement: Restrictions apply to the availability of some or all data generated or analyzed during this study. The corresponding author will on request detail the restrictions and any conditions under which access to some data may be provided.

Acknowledgments: We thank all of the participants for their help with breastfeeding research.

Conflicts of Interest: D.T.G. declares past participation in the Scientific Advisory Board of Medela AG. All authors are/were supported by an unrestricted research grant from Medela AG, administered by The University of Western Australia. The funders had no role in the design of the study; in the collection, analyses or interpretation of data; in the writing of the manuscript or in the decision to publish the results. All other authors declare no conflicts of interest.

References

- Prime, D.K.; Geddes, D.T.; Hepworth, A.R.; Trengove, N.J.; Hartmann, P.E. Comparison of the patterns of milk ejection during repeated breast expression sessions in women. *Breastfeed. Med.* **2011**, *6*, 183–190. [CrossRef] [PubMed]
- Prime, D.K.; Kent, J.C.; Hepworth, A.R.; Trengove, N.J.; Hartmann, P.E. Dynamics of milk removal during simultaneous breast expression in women. *Breastfeed. Med.* **2012**, *7*, 100–106. [CrossRef] [PubMed]

Disclaimer/Publisher's Note: The statements, opinions and data contained in all publications are solely those of the individual author(s) and contributor(s) and not of MDPI and/or the editor(s). MDPI and/or the editor(s) disclaim responsibility for any injury to people or property resulting from any ideas, methods, instructions or products referred to in the content.

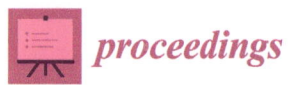

Abstract

GenV: Preservation of Human Milk for Biological Discovery [†]

Ching Tat Lai [1,2,3,*], Kim Powell [4], Yeukai Mangwiro [4], Tony Frugier [4], Anna Fedyukova [4], Jatender Mohal [4], William Siero [4], Sharon L. Perrella [1,2,3], Melissa Wake [4,5], Mary E. Wlodek [4,5,6], Richard Saffery [4,5] and Donna T. Geddes [1,2,3]

[1] School of Molecular Sciences, The University of Western Australia, Perth, WA 6009, Australia; sharon.perrella@uwa.edu.au (S.L.P.); donna.geddes@uwa.edu.au (D.T.G.)
[2] ABREAST Network, Perth, WA 6000, Australia
[3] UWA Centre for Human Lactation Research and Translation, Perth, WA 6009, Australia
[4] Murdoch Children's Research Institute, Royal Children's Hospital, Melbourne, VIC 3052, Australia; kim.powell@mcri.edu.au (K.P.); yeukai.mangwiro@mcri.edu.au (Y.M.); tony.frugier@mcri.edu.au (T.F.); anna.fedyukova@mcri.edu.au (A.F.); jatender.mohal@mcri.edu.au (J.M.); william.siero@mcri.edu.au (W.S.); melissa.wake@mcri.edu.au (M.W.); m.wlodek@unimelb.edu.au (M.E.W.); richard.saffery@mcri.edu.au (R.S.)
[5] Department of Paediatrics, Royal Children's Hospital, Melbourne, VIC 3052, Australia
[6] Department of Obstetrics and Gynaecology, The University of Melbourne, Melbourne, VIC 3010, Australia
* Correspondence: ching-tat.lai@uwa.edu.au
[†] Presented at Australian Breastfeeding + Lactation Research and Science Translation Conference (ABREAST Conference 2024), Perth, Australia, 15 November 2024.

Abstract: Human milk contains a variety of biologically active molecules that are essential for infant growth and development, as well as indicators of maternal health. However understanding the full potential of these molecules is challenging due to variations in their concentrations among mothers, potential degradation during sample handling and storage, and the limited accessibility of specific human milk analyses. This study aimed to evaluate the effectiveness of a freeze-dried preservative cocktail in maintaining the stability of key milk molecules during collection, transport, and storage. GenV participants ($n = 96$) were given a sample collection kit and followed the instructions to collect approximately 5 mL of breast milk, which was placed in a collection tube containing the preservative. The samples were mailed at ambient temperature to the GenV laboratory (Murdoch Children's Research Institute, Melbourne, Victoria, Australia), where they were aliquoted into 1 mL tubes using a liquid handling system (Janus) and stored at −80 °C. These samples were randomly selected and sent to The University of Western Australia (Perth, Western Australia, Australia) on dry ice for biochemical analysis. The average collection day postpartum was 16 ± 14 (range 1–91 days), while the average postal receipt time was 5 ± 3 days (range 1–16 days), and samples were processed within 6 days of receipt (average 3 ± 2 days). The mean concentrations of key molecules—fat (48.6 ± 17.1 g/L), protein (15.5 ± 4.3 g/L), lactose (78.9 ± 13.9 g/L), glucose (0.17 ± 0.17 g/L), lysozyme (0.16 ± 0.16 g/L), and insulin (6.1 ± 4.9 µIU/mL)—were consistent with reported literature values. There were no statistically significant differences in molecular concentrations based on postal transit time, receipt, or processing delays ($p > 0.05$). These results demonstrate that the preservative cocktail effectively preserved the integrity of key molecules in human milk during handling, postal transport, and storage at ambient temperature. The findings support its use as a valuable tool for human milk research, enabling more flexible sample collection and handling without compromising the quality of the milk or the biochemical analysis. Future research should explore its application in broader contexts to further enhance the accuracy and reliability of milk composition studies across diverse research settings.

Keywords: human milk; preservative; storage; handling; GenV

Academic Editors: Nicolas L. Taylor and Debbie Palmer

Published: 2 January 2025

Citation: Lai, C.T.; Powell, K.; Mangwiro, Y.; Frugier, T.; Fedyukova, A.; Mohal, J.; Siero, W.; Perrella, S.L.; Wake, M.; Wlodek, M.E.; et al. GenV: Preservation of Human Milk for Biological Discovery. *Proceedings* **2025**, *112*, 10. https://doi.org/10.3390/proceedings2025112010

Copyright: © 2025 by the authors. Licensee MDPI, Basel, Switzerland. This article is an open access article distributed under the terms and conditions of the Creative Commons Attribution (CC BY) license (https://creativecommons.org/licenses/by/4.0/).

Author Contributions: Conceptualization, C.T.L. and D.T.G.; methodology, C.T.L. and D.T.G.; formal analysis, C.T.L.; investigation, D.T.G. and C.T.L.; resources, D.T.G.; data curation, C.T.L. and D.T.G.; writing—original draft preparation, C.T.L.; writing—review and editing, D.T.G., J.M., A.F., W.S., T.F., K.P., Y.M., S.L.P., M.W., M.E.W. and R.S.; visualization, C.T.L.; supervision, D.T.G.; funding acquisition, D.T.G. All authors have read and agreed to the published version of the manuscript.

Funding: This research was funded by an unrestricted research grant from Medela AG (Switzerland). C.T.L. and D.T.G. receive a salary from an unrestricted research grant paid by Medela AG and administered by The University of Western Australia. The funders had no role in the design of the study; in the collection, analyses, or interpretation of the data; in the writing of the manuscript; or in the decision to publish the results.

Institutional Review Board Statement: This study was conducted in accordance with the Declaration of Helsinki. The study was approved by the Human Research Ethics Committee at The University of Western Australia (2019/RA/4/20/4023) and conducted in accordance with the relevant guidelines and regulations.

Informed Consent Statement: Informed consent was obtained from all subjects involved in the study.

Data Availability Statement: Not applicable.

Acknowledgments: We thank all our participants and their families for their time and help with this research.

Conflicts of Interest: D.T.G. declares participation in the Scientific Advisory Board of Medela AG. C.T.L. and D.T.G. are/were supported by an unrestricted research grant from Medela AG, administered by The University of Western Australia. The funders had no role in the design of the study; in the collection, analyses, or interpretation of the data; in the writing of the manuscript; or in the decision to publish the results. All other authors declare no conflicts of interest.

Disclaimer/Publisher's Note: The statements, opinions and data contained in all publications are solely those of the individual author(s) and contributor(s) and not of MDPI and/or the editor(s). MDPI and/or the editor(s) disclaim responsibility for any injury to people or property resulting from any ideas, methods, instructions or products referred to in the content.

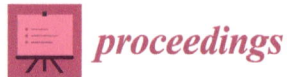 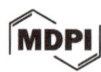

Abstract

Multiple Lactations: Effect of Successive Lactation on Milk Production and Infant Milk Intake [†]

Ashleigh H. Warden [1,2,3], Vanessa S. Sakalidis [4], Jacki L. McEachran [1,2,3], Ching Tat Lai [1,2,3], Sharon L. Perrella [1,2,3], Donna T. Geddes [1,2,3] and Zoya Gridneva [1,2,3,*]

[1] School of Molecular Sciences, The University of Western Australia, Crawley, WA 6009, Australia; asleigh.warden@uwa.edu.au (A.H.W.); jacki.mceachran@uwa.edu.au (J.L.M.); ching-tat.lai@uwa.edu.au (C.T.L.); sharon.perrella@uwa.edu.au (S.L.P.); donna.geddes@uwa.edu.au (D.T.G)
[2] ABREAST Network, Perth, WA 6000, Australia
[3] UWA Centre for Human Lactation Research and Translation, Crawley, WA 6009, Australia
[4] Menzies School of Health Research, Royal Darwin Hospital Campus, Casuarina, NT 0810, Australia; vanessa.sakalidis@menzies.edu.au
[*] Correspondence: zoya.gridneva@uwa.edu.au
[†] Presented at Australian Breastfeeding + Lactation Research and Science Translation Conference (ABREAST Conference 2024), Perth, Australia, 15 November 2024.

Abstract: Optimal infant growth is reliant on both the production and intake of sufficient human milk. Some studies, in particular animal models, suggest that multiparous mothers produce a higher yield of milk compared to primiparous mothers. The aim of this study was to examine whether there is a relationship between successive lactations and maternal 24 h milk production and infant milk intake. Lactating mothers who did not feed commercial milk formula ($n = 22$) measured their milk production at 1–6 months postpartum by test-weighing their infants for 24 h during two consecutive lactations (L1: at 3.0 ± 1.2 months, L2: at 2.6 ± 1.0 months; ($p = 0.26$)) and provided the dyad's demographics. Twenty-four-hour milk production by breast, infant 24 h milk intake (including mothers' own expressed milk), and breastfeeding and expressing frequencies were measured. Statistical analysis used linear mixed modelling accounting for infant birth weight and the random effect of participant. There were no differences between L1 and L2 for milk production (L1: 748 ± 122 g; L2: 768 ± 157 g; $p = 0.57$), infant milk intake (L1: 744 ± 133 g; L2: 776 ± 189 g; $p = 0.50$), 24 h breastfeeding frequency (L1: 13 ± 4; L2: 12 ± 3; $p = 0.28$), and expression frequency (L1: 1.4 ± 1.9; L2: 1.4 ± 2.8; $p = 0.95$). Birth weight was higher with the successive lactation (L1: 3260 ± 345 g; L2: 3509 ± 237 g; $p = 0.002$). Infant sex was not associated with 24 h milk production ($p = 0.21$), milk intake ($p = 0.62$), or breastfeeding frequency ($p = 0.17$). The findings of this study suggest that in humans there is no effect of successive lactations or infant sex on 24 h milk production or infant milk intake.

Keywords: human milk; lactation; milk production; milk intake; successive lactation; infant; early nutrition; birth weight

Author Contributions: Conceptualization, Z.G. and D.T.G.; methodology, Z.G., V.S.S., C.T.L. and S.L.P.; software, V.S.S.; validation, A.H.W., J.L.M. and Z.G.; formal analysis, A.H.W., V.S.S. and Z.G.; investigation, A.H.W. and Z.G.; resources, D.T.G.; data curation, A.H.W., J.L.M., S.L.P. and Z.G.; writing—original draft preparation, A.H.W.; writing—review and editing, V.S.S., J.L.M., C.T.L., S.L.P., D.T.G. and Z.G.; visualization, A.H.W.; supervision, Z.G. and D.T.G.; project administration, J.L.M.; funding acquisition, D.T.G. All authors have read and agreed to the published version of the manuscript.

Funding: This research was funded by an unrestricted research grant from Medela AG (Switzerland). The funder had no role in the design of the study; in the collection, analyses, or interpretation of data; in the writing of the manuscript; or in the decision to publish the results.

Institutional Review Board Statement: The study was conducted in accordance with the Declaration of Helsinki and was approved by The University of Western Australia Human Research Ethics Committee (2019/RA/4/20/6134).

Informed Consent Statement: Informed consent was obtained from all subjects involved in the study.

Data Availability Statement: Restrictions apply to the availability of some or all data generated or analysed during this study. The corresponding author will, on request, detail the restrictions and any conditions under which access to some data may be provided.

Acknowledgments: We thank all of the participants for help with breastfeeding research.

Conflicts of Interest: D.T.G. declares past participation in the Scientific Advisory Board of Medela AG. All authors are/were supported by an unrestricted research grant from Medela AG, administered by The University of Western Australia. The funders had no role in the design of the study; in the collection, analyses, or interpretation of data; in the writing of the manuscript; or in the decision to publish the results. All other authors declare no conflicts of interest.

Disclaimer/Publisher's Note: The statements, opinions and data contained in all publications are solely those of the individual author(s) and contributor(s) and not of MDPI and/or the editor(s). MDPI and/or the editor(s) disclaim responsibility for any injury to people or property resulting from any ideas, methods, instructions or products referred to in the content.

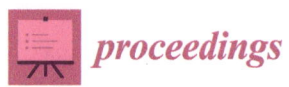

Abstract

Impact of Diet on the Maternal and Infant Microbiota [†]

Donna T. Geddes [1,2,3,*], Azhar S. Sindi [1,2,3,4], Ching Tat Lai [1,2,3], Zoya Gridneva [1,2,3], Gabriela E. Leghi [5], Mary E. Wlodek [1,6], Lisa F. Stinson [1,2,3], Xiaojie Zhou [1,2,3], Matthew S. Payne [7], Merryn J. Netting [6,8,9], Michelle L. Trevenen [10], Alethea Rea [10,11] and Beverly S. Muhlhausler [5,12]

1. School of Molecular Sciences, The University of Western Australia, Perth, WA 6009, Australia; asmsindi@uqu.edu.sa (A.S.S.); ching-tat.lai@uwa.edu.au (C.T.L.); zoya.gridneva@uwa.edu.au (Z.G.); m.wlodek@unimelb.edu.au (M.E.W.); lisa.stinson@uwa.edu.au (L.F.S.); xiaojie.zhou@uwa.edu.au (X.Z.)
2. ABREAST Network, Perth, WA 6000, Australia
3. UWA Centre for Human Lactation Research and Translation, Perth, WA 6009, Australia
4. College of Applied Medical Sciences, Umm Al-Qura University, Makkah 24381-8156, Saudi Arabia
5. School of Agriculture, Food and Wine, The University of Adelaide, Adelaide, SA 5064, Australia; gabriela.leghivoyer@gmail.com (G.E.L.); bev.muhlhausler@csiro.au (B.S.M.)
6. Department of Obstetrics and Gynaecology, University of Melbourne, Melbourne, VIC 3010, Australia; merryn.netting@sahmri.com
7. Division of Obstetrics and Gynaecology, School of Medicine, The University of Western Australia, Perth, WA 6009, Australia; matthew.payne@uwa.edu.au
8. Discipline of Paediatrics, The University of Adelaide, Adelaide, SA 5006, Australia
9. Women's and Children's Hospital, Adelaide, SA 5006, Australia
10. Centre for Applied Statistics, The University of Western Australia, Perth, WA 6009, Australia; michelle.trevenen@uwa.edu.au (M.L.T.); alethea.rea@murdoch.edu.au (A.R.)
11. Mathematics and Statistics, Murdoch University, Murdoch, WA 6150, Australia
12. CSIRO, Adelaide, SA 5000, Australia
* Correspondence: donna.geddes@uwa.edu.au
† Presented at Australian Breastfeeding + Lactation Research and Science Translation Conference (ABREAST Conference 2024), Perth, Australia, 15 November 2024.

Keywords: breastfeeding; lactation; human milk; diet; body composition; milk composition; microbiome; infants

Whilst diet plays a pivotal role in human health, very little research on the lactation period exists. Research studying the influence of maternal nutrition on maternal health, milk composition and infant health provides conflicting results [1]. It is often hypothesized that the maternal diet influences the maternal condition (e.g., microbiome and body composition), which in turn influences milk composition (e.g., microbiome, macronutrients, hormones, and immune proteins) and then impacts the infant (e.g., gut microbiome). We conducted a within-participant intervention, where maternal meals with reduced fat and sugar and increased fiber were provided for 2 weeks after a 1-week dietary monitoring period. Shotgun metagenomic sequencing of stool samples from 10 infants (n = 20, one sample pre-diet and one post-diet) revealed no differences in the microbiome composition. However, changes in maternal fiber, sugar and fat intake were associated with changes in the functional potential of the infant gut microbiome [2]. To determine changes in the maternal gut microbiome in response to the dietary intervention and subsequently the human milk microbiome, we analyzed fecal swabs and milk samples collected from 11 mothers prior to the intervention, post-intervention, and 4 and 8 weeks post intervention. Small but significant changes were found in the relative abundance of two fecal bacteria immediately post intervention: *Bacteroides caccae* (decreased) and *Faecalibacillus intestinalis* (increased) however, seven bacteria changed in the 4 to 8 weeks post intervention. Similarly, the abundance of two bacteria changed in human milk; *Cutibacterium acnes* increased and

Haemophilus parainfluenzae decreased. Two additional human milk bacteria differed in the 4-to-8-week intervention follow-up period [3]. Interestingly, we found no differences in the macronutrient content in the daily human milk samples across the full 3-week period [4]. Conversely, after the dietary intervention, the insulin, leptin and adiponectin concentrations in human milk were decreased by 10–25%. This is likely due to the significant reduction in the maternal body weight (−1.8%) and fat mass (−6.3%). Analysis of the immune proteins lactoferrin and lysozyme in daily milk samples across the 3-week study period showed a relatively small but significant decrease in lactoferrin. This may reflect an improved maternal inflammatory status [5]. Further, the short-term diet had no effects on 24 h milk production or infant growth [6].

Author Contributions: Conceptualization, D.T.G., B.S.M., M.E.W. and L.F.S.; methodology, B.S.M., M.S.P., D.T.G., C.T.L., L.F.S., M.J.N., A.R., M.L.T., G.E.L. and A.S.S.; data collection, G.E.L.; formal analysis, C.T.L.; investigation, C.T.L., L.F.S., Z.G., X.Z. and D.T.G.; resources, D.T.G., M.J.N., A.R. and M.L.T.; data curation, G.E.L. and A.S.S.; writing—original draft preparation, D.T.G.; writing—review and editing, B.S.M., M.S.P., D.T.G., C.T.L., L.F.S., Z.G., X.Z., M.J.N., A.R., M.L.T., G.E.L., A.S.S., C.T.L., M.E.W. and L.F.S.; supervision, C.T.L., L.F.S., B.S.M., M.E.W. and D.T.G.; project administration, D.T.G.; funding acquisition, B.S.M. and D.T.G. All authors have read and agreed to the published version of the manuscript.

Funding: This research was funded by unrestricted research grant from Medela AG (Switzerland) administered by The University of Western Australia. The funders had no role in the design of the study; in the collection, analyses, or interpretation of data; in the writing of the manuscript; or in the decision to publish the results.

Institutional Review Board Statement: The study was conducted in accordance with the Declaration of Helsinki. The study was approved by the Human Research Ethics Committee at The University of Western Australia (RA/4/20/4953) and conducted in accordance with the relevant guidelines and regulations.

Informed Consent Statement: Informed consent was obtained from all participating mothers at enrollment.

Data Availability Statement: Restrictions apply to the availability of some, or all data generated or analyzed during this study. The corresponding author will, on request, detail the restrictions and any conditions under which access to some data may be provided.

Conflicts of Interest: D.T.G. declares past participation in the Scientific Advisory Board of Medela C.T.L., L.F.S., Z.G., X.J. and D.T.G are/were supported by an unrestricted research grant from Medela AG, administered by The University of Western Australia. The funders had no role in the design of the study; in the collection, analyses, or interpretation of data; in the writing of the manuscript; or in the decision to publish the results.

References

1. Sindi, A.S.; Geddes, D.T.; Wlodek, M.E.; Muhlhausler, B.S.; Payne, M.S.; Stinson, L.F. Can we modulate the breastfed infant gut microbiota through maternal diet? *FEMS Microbiol. Rev.* **2021**, *45*, fuab011. [CrossRef] [PubMed]
2. Sindi, A.S.; Stinson, L.F.; Lean, S.S.; Chooi, Y.H.; Leghi, G.E.; Netting, M.J.; Wlodek, M.E.; Muhlhausler, B.S.; Geddes, D.T.; Payne, M.S. Effect of a reduced fat and sugar maternal dietary intervention during lactation on the infant gut microbiome. *Front. Microbiol.* **2022**, *13*, 900702. [CrossRef] [PubMed]
3. Sindi, A.S.; Stinson, L.F.; Gridneva, Z.; Leghi, G.E.; Netting, M.J.; Wlodek, M.E.; Muhlhausler, B.S.; Rea, A.; Trevenen, M.L.; Geddes, D.T.; et al. Maternal dietary intervention during lactation impacts the maternal faecal and human milk microbiota. *J. Appl. Microbiol.* **2024**, *135*, lxae024. [CrossRef]
4. Leghi, G.E.; Lai, C.T.; Narayanan, A.; Netting, M.J.; Dymock, M.; Rea, A.; Wlodek, M.E.; Geddes, D.T.; Muhlhausler, B.S. Daily variation of macronutrient concentrations in mature human milk over 3 weeks. *Sci. Rep.* **2021**, *11*, 10224. [CrossRef]

5. Sindi, A.S.; Stinson, L.F.; Lai, C.T.; Gridneva, Z.; Leghi, G.E.; Netting, M.J.; Wlodek, M.E.; Muhlhausler, B.S.; Zhou, X.; Payne, M.S.; et al. Human milk lactoferrin and lysozyme concentrations vary in response to a dietary intervention. *J. Nutr. Biochem.* **2024**, *135*, 109760. [CrossRef] [PubMed]
6. Leghi, G.E.; Netting, M.J.; Lai, C.T.; Narayanan, A.; Dymock, M.; Rea, A.; Wlodek, M.E.; Geddes, D.T.; Muhlhausler, B.S. Reduction in maternal energy intake during lactation decreased maternal body weight and concentrations of leptin, insulin and adiponectin in human milk without affecting milk production, milk macronutrient composition or infant growth. *Nutrients* **2021**, *13*, 1892. [CrossRef] [PubMed]

Disclaimer/Publisher's Note: The statements, opinions and data contained in all publications are solely those of the individual author(s) and contributor(s) and not of MDPI and/or the editor(s). MDPI and/or the editor(s) disclaim responsibility for any injury to people or property resulting from any ideas, methods, instructions or products referred to in the content.

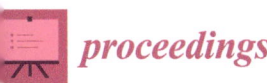

Abstract

Breastfeeding, Human Milk and Allergic Disease: Findings from the CHILD Cohort Study [†]

Meghan B. Azad [1,2]

1 Manitoba Interdisciplinary Lactation Centre (MILC), Children's Hospital Research Institute of Manitoba, Winnipeg, MB R3E 3P4, Canada; meghan.azad@umanitoba.ca
2 Department of Pediatrics and Child Health, University of Manitoba, Winnipeg, MB R3T 2N2, Canada
† Presented at Australian Breastfeeding + Lactation Research and Science Translation Conference (ABREAST Conference 2024), Perth, Australia, 15 November 2024.

Keywords: breastfeeding; human milk; allergic disease; asthma; food allergy; microbiome; immunity; CHILD Cohort Study

Breastfeeding substantially contributes to infant microbiome and immune development, influencing lifelong health trajectories, including allergic disease risk. However, the nuances of these relationships and underlying mechanisms are not fully understood. The CHILD Cohort Study (www.childstudy.ca) follows 3500 Canadian families from pregnancy through adolescence to understand the developmental origins of asthma, allergies, and other chronic health conditions. Within CHILD, infant feeding practices (e.g., exclusivity, duration, and mode of human milk feeding) and human milk composition (e.g., microbiota, oligosaccharides, nutrients, and bioactive proteins) are studied to understand their contributions to infant microbiome development and health. CHILD findings show that breastfeeding shapes infant microbiome development [1–4] and serum immune biomarker profiles in the first year of life [5]. Breastfeeding appears to protect against childhood asthma in a dose-dependent manner that is strongest with direct nursing (vs. feeding pumped breastmilk) [6] and partially mediated through the nasal and gut microbiomes [7]. The combination of maternal peanut consumption and breastfeeding at the time of peanut introduction during infancy is associated with a lower risk of peanut sensitization through 5 years of age [8]. Using approaches to interrogate human milk as a complex biological system (rather than discrete individual components) [9,10], allergic disease phenotypes have been associated with specific combinations of human milk oligosaccharides [11], polyunsaturated fatty acids [12], and microbiota [13,14]. In conclusion, the CHILD Cohort Study has identified infant feeding practices, human milk components, and related biological mechanisms that may contribute to the development or prevention of allergic phenotypes. Expansion of this research could identify new therapeutic targets and disease prevention strategies.

Funding: M.B.A. holds a Canada Research Chair in Early Nutrition and the Developmental Origins of Health and Disease and is a fellow of the CIFAR Humans and the Microbiome Program. The CHILD Cohort Study was established with funding from the Canadian Institutes of Health Research and the Allergy, Genes, and Environment Network of Centres of Excellence. The analysis of CHILD samples and data, for the studies summarized here, was funded by a variety of sources, each listed in the cited publications.

Institutional Review Board Statement: CHILD Cohort Study protocols were approved by the Human Research Ethics Boards at McMaster University, the Hospital for Sick Children, and the Universities of Manitoba, Alberta, and British Columbia.

Informed Consent Statement: Informed consent was obtained from all participating mothers at enrollment.

Data Availability Statement: CHILD Study data are available by registration to the CHILD database (https://childstudy.ca/childdb/) and the submission of a formal request.

Acknowledgments: We thank the CHILD Cohort Study (CHILD) participant families for their dedication and commitment to advancing health research.

Conflicts of Interest: M.B.A. has consulted for DSM Nutritional Products, serves on the scientific advisory board for TinyHealth, and has received speaking honoraria from Prolacta Biosciences. She has contributed without remuneration to online courses on breast milk and the infant microbiome produced by Microbiome Courses. For all research summarized here, funders had no role in the design of the study; in the collection, analyses, or interpretation of data; in the writing of the manuscript; or in the decision to publish the results.

References

1. Dai, D.L.Y.; Petersen, C.; Hoskinson, C.; Del Bel, K.L.; Becker, A.B.; Moraes, T.J.; Mandhane, P.J.; Finlay, B.B.; Simons, E.; Kozyrskyj, A.L.; et al. Breastfeeding enrichment of B. longum subsp. infantis mitigates the effect of antibiotics on the microbiota and childhood asthma risk. *Med* **2023**, *4*, 92–112.e5. [CrossRef]
2. Fehr, K.; Moossavi, S.; Sbihi, H.; Boutin, R.C.T.; Bode, L.; Robertson, B.; Yonemitsu, C.; Field, C.J.; Becker, A.B.; Mandhane, P.J.; et al. Breastmilk feeding practices are associated with the co-occurrence of bacteria in mothers' milk and the infant gut: The CHILD Cohort Study. *Cell Host Microbe* **2020**, *28*, 285–297.e4. [CrossRef] [PubMed]
3. Forbes, J.D.; Azad, M.B.; Vehling, L.; Tun, H.M.; Konya, T.B.; Guttman, D.S.; Field, C.J.; Lefebvre, D.; Sears, M.R.; Becker, A.B.; et al. Association of exposure to formula in the hospital and subsequent infant feeding practices with gut microbiota and risk of overweight in the first year of life. *JAMA Pediatr.* **2018**, *172*, e181161. [CrossRef] [PubMed]
4. Azad, M.B.; Konya, T.; Maughan, H.; Guttman, D.S.; Field, C.J.; Chari, R.S.; Sears, M.R.; Becker, A.B.; Scott, J.A.; Kozyrskyj, A.L.; et al. Gut microbiota of healthy Canadian infants: Profiles by mode of delivery and infant diet at 4 months. *CMAJ* **2013**, *185*, 385–394. [CrossRef] [PubMed]
5. Ames, S.R.; Lotoski, L.C.; Rodriguez, L.; Brodin, P.; Mandhane, P.J.; Moraes, T.J.; Simons, E.; Turvey, S.E.; Subbarao, P.; Azad, M.B. Human milk feeding practices and serum immune profiles of one-year-old infants in the CHILD birth cohort study. *Am. J. Clin. Nutr.* **2025**, *121*, 60–73. [CrossRef] [PubMed]
6. Klopp, A.; Vehling, L.; Becker, A.B.; Subbarao, P.; Mandhane, P.J.; Turvey, S.E.; Lefebvre, D.L.; Sears, M.R.; CHILD Study Investigators; Azad, M.B. Modes of infant feeding and the risk of childhood asthma: A prospective birth cohort study. *J. Pediatr.* **2017**, *190*, 192–199.e2. [CrossRef] [PubMed]
7. Shenhav, L.; Fehr, K.; Reyna, M.E.; Petersen, C.; Dai, D.L.Y.; Dai, R.; Breton, V.; Rossi, L.; Smieja, M.; Simons, E.; et al. Microbial colonization programs are structured by breastfeeding and guide healthy respiratory development. *Cell* **2024**, *187*, 5431–5452.e20. [CrossRef]
8. Azad, M.B.; Dharma, C.; Simons, E.; Tran, M.; Reyna, M.E.; Dai, R.; Becker, A.B.; Marshall, J.; Mandhane, P.J.; Turvey, S.E.; et al. Reduced peanut sensitization with maternal peanut consumption and early peanut introduction while breastfeeding. *J. Dev. Orig. Health Dis.* **2021**, *12*, 811–818. [CrossRef]
9. Shenhav, L.; Azad, M.B. Using community ecology theory and computational microbiome methods to study human milk as a biological system. *mSystems* **2022**, *7*, e01132-21. [CrossRef] [PubMed]
10. Becker, M.; Fehr, K.; Goguen, S.; Miliku, K.; Field, C.; Robertson, B.; Yonemitsu, C.; Bode, L.; Simons, E.; Marshall, J.; et al. Multimodal machine learning for modeling infant head circumference, mothers' milk composition, and their shared environment. *Sci. Rep.* **2024**, *14*, 2977. [CrossRef] [PubMed]
11. Miliku, K.; Robertson, B.; Sharma, A.K.; Subbarao, P.; Becker, A.B.; Mandhane, P.J.; Turvey, S.E.; Lefebvre, D.L.; Sears, M.R.; CHILD Study Investigators; et al. Human milk oligosaccharide profiles and food sensitization among infants in the CHILD Study. *Allergy* **2018**, *73*, 2070–2073. [CrossRef] [PubMed]
12. Miliku, K.; Richelle, J.; Becker, A.B.; Simons, E.; Moraes, T.J.; Stuart, T.E.; Mandhane, P.J.; Sears, M.R.; Subbarao, P.; Field, C.J.; et al. Sex-specific associations of human milk long-chain polyunsaturated fatty acids and infant allergic conditions. *Pediatr. Allergy Immunol.* **2021**, *32*, 1173–1182. [CrossRef] [PubMed]

13. Fang, Z.Y.; Stickley, S.A.; Ambalavanan, A.; Zhang, Y.; Zacharias, A.M.; Fehr, K.; Moossavi, S.; Petersen, C.; Miliku, K.; Mandhane, P.J.; et al. Networks of human milk microbiota are associated with host genomics, childhood asthma, and allergic sensitization. *Cell Host Microbe* **2024**, *32*, 1838–1852.e5. [CrossRef] [PubMed]
14. Ambalavanan, A.; Chang, L.; Choi, J.; Zhang, Y.; Stickley, S.A.; Fang, Z.Y.; Miliku, K.; Robertson, B.; Yonemitsu, C.; Turvey, S.E.; et al. Human milk oligosaccharides are associated with maternal genetics and respiratory health of human milk-fed children. *Nat. Commun.* **2024**, *15*, 7735. [CrossRef] [PubMed]

Disclaimer/Publisher's Note: The statements, opinions and data contained in all publications are solely those of the individual author(s) and contributor(s) and not of MDPI and/or the editor(s). MDPI and/or the editor(s) disclaim responsibility for any injury to people or property resulting from any ideas, methods, instructions or products referred to in the content.

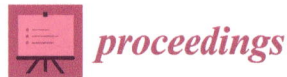
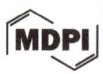

Abstract

Pain Ratings and Pharmacological Pain Management in Australian Breastfeeding Women After a Caesarean Section Birth [†]

Jasmine E. Hunt [1,2], Philip Vlaskovsky [3], Ching T. Lai [2,4,5], Sarah G. Abelha [2,4,5], Jacki L. McEachran [2,4,5], Stuart A. Prosser [2,6], Donna T. Geddes [2,4,5] and Sharon L. Perrella [2,4,5,*]

1. School of Medicine, The University of Western Australia, Crawley, WA 6009, Australia; 22969223@student.uwa.edu.au
2. School of Molecular Sciences, The University of Western Australia, Crawley, WA 6009, Australia; ching-tat.lai@uwa.edu.au (C.T.L.); sarah.abelha@uwa.edu.au (S.G.A.); jacki.mceachran@uwa.edu.au (J.L.M.); stuart@westernobs.com.au (S.A.P.); donna.geddes@uwa.edu.au (D.T.G.)
3. School of Mathematics and Statistics, The University of Western Australia, Crawley, WA 6009, Australia; philip.vlaskovsky@uwa.edu.au
4. ABREAST Network, Perth, WA 6000, Australia
5. UWA Centre for Human Lactation Research and Translation, Crawley, WA 6009, Australia
6. Western Obstetrics, Balcatta, WA 6021, Australia
* Correspondence: sharon.perrella@uwa.edu.au; Tel.: +61-6488-1208
[†] Presented at Australian Breastfeeding + Lactation Research and Science Translation Conference (ABREAST Conference 2024), Perth, Australia, 15 November 2024.

Keywords: caesarean section; pain; analgesia; obstetrical; postpartum period; analgesics; opioid; anaesthesia

Academic Editors: Nicolas L. Taylor and Debbie Palmer

Published: 7 January 2025

Citation: Hunt, J.E.; Vlaskovsky, P.; Lai, C.T.; Abelha, S.G.; McEachran, J.L.; Prosser, S.A.; Geddes, D.T.; Perrella, S.L. Pain Ratings and Pharmacological Pain Management in Australian Breastfeeding Women After a Caesarean Section Birth. *Proceedings* 2025, *112*, 14. https://doi.org/10.3390/proceedings2025112014

Copyright: © 2025 by the authors. Licensee MDPI, Basel, Switzerland. This article is an open access article distributed under the terms and conditions of the Creative Commons Attribution (CC BY) license (https://creativecommons.org/licenses/by/4.0/).

Caesarean section (CS) birth is associated with pain and reduced mobility that impacts a woman's ability to breastfeed and care for her newborn infant. Post-CS pain, difficulties in mobilising and medication side effects pose challenges to picking up the infant and breastfeeding; these factors may contribute to lower rates of exclusive or any breastfeeding after CS birth. Anaesthetic type, postpartum pain levels and use of analgesia differ between women after CS. A better understanding of post-CS pain and analgesia use is needed to optimise maternal comfort and safety of the breastfeeding dyad in the postpartum period. We analysed an existing dataset of $n = 824$ online anonymous survey responses from Australian women who gave birth via CS within the previous 12 months [1]. Participants provided details of their CS birth and breastfeeding experiences, pain ratings (range 0–10) in the hours and days after birth and in the first two weeks after discharge and post-discharge analgesia use. The aim of this secondary analysis was to determine early postpartum maternal pain scores and analgesia use after CS birth. We also explored associations between biopsychosocial factors, pain scores and post-discharge analgesia use.

Descriptive statistics were used to summarise postpartum pain ratings and analgesia use in the first two weeks after hospital discharge. Linear mixed model and linear regression tested for associations between biopsychosocial factors and pain scores over time, and pain in the first two weeks after discharge, respectively. Logistic regression models were used to investigate associations with opioid consumption and the duration of non-opioid analgesia use after discharge. Median (Q1, Q3) pain scores were 3 (1, 6) in the early hours and 6 (4, 8) in the first few days after birth, and 5 (3, 7) in the first two weeks after discharge. Participants who had a non-elective lower uterine segment CS (NELUSCS) reported higher pain scores in the first few days after birth ($\beta = 0.40$; 95% CI 0.01, 0.79; $p = 0.043$) and in the first two weeks after discharge ($\beta = 0.67$; 95% CI 0.28, 1.07; $p < 0.001$) when compared to those who had an elective lower uterine segment CS (ELUSCS). Unmet birth expectations (β = 0.60; 95% CI 0.15, 1.06; p = 0.010) and birth trauma (β = 0.55; 95% CI 0.09, 1.00; p = 0.020) were also associated with higher pain scores in the first two weeks after discharge in the marginal model; however, NELUSCS was no longer significant (β = −0.06; 95% CI −0.52, 0.40; p = 0.79). CS birth at a private hospital was associated with lower pain scores in the first two weeks after discharge (β = −0.76; 95% CI −1.11, −0.41; p < 0.001). Most participants used paracetamol (95.8%) and NSAIDs (81.9%), while over half used at least one type of opioid analgesia in the first two weeks after discharge (ELUSCS: 62.3%, NELUSCS: 65.4%). Higher early postpartum pain ratings were associated with greater odds of opioid use after discharge (OR = 1.15; 95% CI 1.06, 1.23; p < 0.001), and an interaction effect was observed between CS type and hospital setting, with NELUSCS at private hospitals associated with increased odds of opioid consumption after discharge (OR = 2.48; 95% CI 1.25, 5.01; p < 0.001). NELUSCS was associated with a longer duration of paracetamol consumption after discharge (OR = 1.38, 95% CI 1.07, 1.80, p = 0.015).

Postpartum pain and analgesia use is higher after NELUSCS birth, indicating the need for the refinement of enhanced recovery after caesarean (ERAC) protocols to improve maternal and breastfeeding outcomes after an unplanned CS birth. Furthermore, psychosocial factors may explain differences in postpartum pain and warrant further investigation. The optimisation of pain management may include using interventions before and after CS birth, with the additional benefit of reducing opioid consumption in line with recommended opioid stewardship practices to minimise risks to the breastfeeding dyad.

Author Contributions: Conceptualization, S.L.P., S.G.A., S.A.P. and D.T.G.; methodology, S.L.P., P.V. and J.E.H.; software, J.L.M.; formal analysis, J.E.H., C.T.L. and P.V.; investigation, S.G.A., J.E.H. and S.L.P.; resources, D.T.G.; data curation, J.L.M.; writing—original draft preparation, J.E.H.; writing—review and editing, P.V., S.G.A., J.L.M., D.T.G. and S.L.P.; supervision, D.T.G. and S.L.P.; project administration, J.L.M.; funding acquisition, D.T.G. All authors have read and agreed to the published version of the manuscript.

Funding: This research was funded by an unrestricted research grant from Medela AG (Switzerland). The funder had no role in the design of the study; in the collection, analyses, or interpretation of data; in the writing of the manuscript; or in the decision to publish the results.

Institutional Review Board Statement: The study was conducted in accordance with the Declaration of Helsinki. The study was approved by the Human Research Ethics Committee at the University of Western Australia (2022/ET000174) and conducted in accordance with the relevant guidelines and regulations.

Informed Consent Statement: Informed consent was obtained from all subjects involved in the study.

Data Availability Statement: Restrictions apply to the availability of some, or all data generated or analysed during this study. The corresponding author will on request detail the restrictions and any conditions under which access to some data may be provided.

Acknowledgments: We thank all of the participants for their help with this research.

Conflicts of Interest: D.T.G. declares past participation in the Scientific Advisory Board of Medela S.G.A., J.L.M., C.T.L., D.T.G. and S.L.P. are supported by an unrestricted research grant from Medela AG, administered by the University of Western Australia. The funder had no role in the design of the study; in the collection, analyses, or interpretation of data; in the writing of the manuscript; or in the decision to publish the results. All other authors declare no conflicts of interest.

Reference

1. Perrella, S.L.; Abelha, S.G.; Vlaskovsky, P.; McEachran, J.L.; Prosser, S.A.; Geddes, D.T. Australian Women's Experiences of Establishing Breastfeeding after Caesarean Birth. *Int. J. Environ. Res. Public Health* **2024**, *21*, 296. [CrossRef]

Disclaimer/Publisher's Note: The statements, opinions and data contained in all publications are solely those of the individual author(s) and contributor(s) and not of MDPI and/or the editor(s). MDPI and/or the editor(s) disclaim responsibility for any injury to people or property resulting from any ideas, methods, instructions or products referred to in the content.

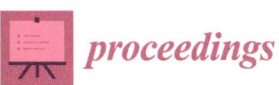

Abstract

Sources and Helpfulness of Breastfeeding Information and Support Accessed by Australian Women Before and After Caesarean Birth [†]

Sarah G. Abelha [1,2,3], Gloria Cheng [4,5], Jacki L. McEachran [1,2,3], Stuart A. Prosser [1,6], Diane L. Spatz [4,7], Donna T. Geddes [1,2,3] and Sharon L. Perrella [1,2,3,6,*]

1. School of Molecular Sciences, The University of Western Australia, Crawley, WA 6009, Australia; sarah.abelha@uwa.edu.au (S.G.A.); jacki.mceachran@uwa.edu.au (J.L.M.); stuart@westernobs.com.au (S.A.P.); donna.geddes@uwa.edu.au (D.T.G.)
2. ABREAST Network, Perth, WA 6000, Australia
3. UWA Centre for Human Lactation Research and Translation, Crawley, WA 6009, Australia
4. School of Nursing, The University of Pennsylvania, Philadelphia, PA 19104, USA; glocheng@wharton.upenn.edu (G.C.); spatz@nursing.upenn.edu (D.L.S.)
5. The Wharton School, The University of Pennsylvania, Philadelphia, PA 19104, USA
6. Western Obstetrics, Balcatta, WA 6021, Australia
7. Centre for Pediatric Nursing Research & Evidence Based Practice, Children's Hospital of Philadelphia, Philadelphia, PA 19104, USA
* Correspondence: sharon.perrella@uwa.edu.au; Tel.: +61-64881208
† Presented at Australian Breastfeeding + Lactation Research and Science Translation Conference (ABREAST Conference 2024), Perth, Australia, 15 November 2024.

Keywords: caesarean section; breastfeeding; education; support; antenatal; postpartum; midwifery; obstetrics

Caesarean section (CS) birth is associated with higher rates of breastfeeding difficulty and has an increasing prevalence in Australia and globally. Therefore, it is important that breastfeeding education and support are optimized to support this group of women. Knowledge of breastfeeding resources accessed by women after CS births and ratings of their helpfulness can inform clinical care and maternal education. The aims of this study were to investigate the prevalence of access and perceived satisfaction with breastfeeding information and support services accessed before and after CS births. Secondary analysis was performed on data from an Australian study that aimed to understand women's experiences of establishing breastfeeding after CS birth. Ref. [1] Women who gave birth via CS within the previous 12 months completed an anonymous online questionnaire that included questions relating to elements of breastfeeding information and care accessed during pregnancy, during the hospital stay and in the first two weeks at home. For the latter period, participants rated the helpfulness of each accessed source using a Likert scale which ranged from 'very helpful' and 'helpful' to 'unsure', 'unhelpful', and 'very unhelpful' or 'not accessed'. A source was deemed helpful if 'helpful' or 'very helpful' had been selected. The sample consisted of 851 women, of which 435 (51.5%) were primiparous. Participants were 5.3 ± 3.6 months postpartum at the time of survey completion, with $n = 689$ (81%) still breastfeeding at that time; the remainder had stopped breastfeeding at 3.2 ± 2.8 months postpartum. There was a balanced representation of women who gave birth in public ($n = 432$, 51%) and private ($n = 419$, 49%) hospitals.

During pregnancy, the most commonly accessed sources of breastfeeding information were midwife (50%), online information (42%), and social media (36%). Half of the primiparous women accessed an antenatal breastfeeding class compared to just 13% of multiparous mothers, and 23% of multiparous women indicated that they did not access any of the listed breastfeeding information sources. Differences in antenatal access to breastfeeding information also differed by health care provider model; women who utilized a private care model were more likely to access an international board-certified lactation consultant (IBCLC) and obstetrician, while women who accessed public care were more likely to access a midwife.

During the postpartum hospital stay, overall, 77% of women accessed a midwife, 41% accessed an IBCLC, and 4% accessed their doctor for breastfeeding support. Compared to multiparous women, primiparous women were more likely to seek support (midwife: 88% vs. 66%, $p < 0.001$; IBCLC 54% vs. 28%, $p < 0.001$). Women who had a non-elective CS birth were more likely to seek breastfeeding support than those who had an elective CS birth (midwife: 83% vs. 73%, $p > 0.001$; IBCLC 47% vs. 37%, $p = 0.003$). Considering healthcare models, 52% of women utilizing private care obtained support from an IBCLC in hospital compared to 32% of those utilizing public maternity care.

In the first two weeks after discharge from hospital, the main sources of breastfeeding support accessed were the partner (97%), child health nurse (77%), and home visiting midwife (68%), while social media was accessed by 54%. Women who had a non-elective CS were more likely to access the home-visiting midwife than those who had an elective CS (73% vs. 64%, $p = 0.007$). Overall access and maternal satisfaction for social, professional, and community-based sources of breastfeeding support were highest for partner, hospital midwife, and IBCLC, respectively. Interestingly, the helpfulness of social media (78%) and midwifery support (hospital 81%, home visiting 79%) were similarly highly rated. The sources most frequently rated as unhelpful were the obstetrician (30%), paediatrician (42%), and Health Direct helpline (28%). Women who utilized private healthcare were more likely to access paid sources of support such as the obstetrician (64% vs. 33%, $p < 0.001$), paediatrician (48% vs. 21%, $p < 0.001$), and community-based IBCLC (58% vs. 46%, $p < 0.001$) for breastfeeding support compared to those utilizing public healthcare.

Women accessed a variety of breastfeeding information and support sources during pregnancy, the hospital stay and in the first few weeks at home, with greater access observed after a non-elective CS birth and in primiparous women. Across all time periods, the most commonly accessed sources of breastfeeding support were midwives and IBCLCs. While ideally placed to support breastfeeding, these sources vary widely with regard to continuity of care, adequacy of time for care provision, and availability of IBCLC services. Depending on healthcare facility staffing, staff workloads, and costs associated with private services, professional breastfeeding support is not readily or evenly accessible for all women. Obstetricians and paediatricians are present immediately after birth and in the early postpartum days, so they are well placed to influence breastfeeding. Given the participants' low ratings of their helpfulness, professional education on lactation and breastfeeding is encouraged for medical staff working in maternity care settings. Online sources and social media were widely accessed and should be utilised by healthcare providers to engage women and their partners in accurate, evidence-based breastfeeding information.

Author Contributions: Conceptualisation, S.L.P., S.G.A. and D.T.G.; methodology, S.L.P., S.G.A., S.A.P. and J.L.M.; software, J.L.M.; formal analysis, G.C., S.G.A. and S.L.P.; investigation, S.G.A. and S.L.P.; resources, D.T.G.; data curation, J.L.M.; writing—original draft preparation, S.G.A.; writing—review and editing, G.C., S.L.P., J.L.M. and D.T.G.; supervision, D.T.G., S.L.P. and D.L.S.; project administration, J.L.M.; funding acquisition, D.T.G. All authors have read and agreed to the published version of the manuscript.

Funding: This research was funded by an unrestricted research grant from Medela AG (Switzerland). The funder had no role in the design of the study; in the collection, analyses, or interpretation of data; in the writing of the manuscript; or in the decision to publish the results.

Institutional Review Board Statement: The study was conducted in accordance with the Declaration of Helsinki. The study was approved by the Human Research Ethics Committee at The University of Western Australia (2022/ET000174) and conducted in accordance with the relevant guidelines and regulations.

Informed Consent Statement: Informed consent was obtained from all subjects involved in the study.

Data Availability Statement: The data that supports the findings of this study is available from the corresponding author upon reasonable request.

Acknowledgments: We would like to thank all the study participants for their generosity and involvement in this study.

Conflicts of Interest: D.T.G. declares past participation in the Scientific Advisory Board of Medela. S.G.A., J.L.M., D.T.G. and S.L.P. are supported by an unrestricted research grant from Medela AG, administered by The University of Western Australia. The funder had no role in the design of the study; in the collection, analyses, or interpretation of data; in the writing of the manuscript; or in the decision to publish the results. All other authors declare no conflicts of interest.

Reference

Perrella, S.L.; Abelha, S.G.; Vlaskovsky, P.; McEachran, J.L.; Prosser, S.A.; Geddes, D.T. Australian Women's Experiences of Establishing Breastfeeding after Caesarean Birth. *Int. J. Environ. Res. Public Health* **2024**, *21*, 296. [CrossRef] [PubMed]

Disclaimer/Publisher's Note: The statements, opinions and data contained in all publications are solely those of the individual author(s) and contributor(s) and not of MDPI and/or the editor(s). MDPI and/or the editor(s) disclaim responsibility for any injury to people or property resulting from any ideas, methods, instructions or products referred to in the content.

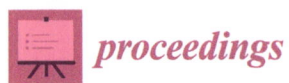

Abstract

Early Feeding Patterns After Pregnancies Complicated by Gestational Diabetes Mellitus [†]

Sharon L. Perrella [1,2,3,4,*], Jacki L. McEachran [1,2,3], Mary E. Wlodek [1,5], Stuart A. Prosser [1,4] and Donna T. Geddes [1,2,3]

[1] School of Molecular Sciences, The University of Western Australia, Crawley, WA 6009, Australia; jacki.mceachran@uwa.edu.au (J.L.M.); m.wlodek@unimelb.edu.au (M.E.W.); stuart@westernobs.com.au (S.A.P.); donna.geddes@uwa.edu.au (D.T.G.)
[2] ABREAST Network, Perth, WA 6000, Australia
[3] UWA Centre for Human Lactation Research and Translation, Crawley, WA 6009, Australia
[4] Western Obstetrics, Balcatta, WA 6021, Australia
[5] Department of Obstetrics and Gynaecology, University of Melbourne, Parkville, VIC 3052, Australia
* Correspondence: sharon.perrella@uwa.edu.au; Tel.: +61-6488-1208
[†] Presented at Australian Breastfeeding + Lactation Research and Science Translation Conference (ABREAST Conference 2024), Perth, Australia, 15 November 2024.

Abstract: Gestational diabetes mellitus (GDM) has been associated with suboptimal breast feeding outcomes, including low milk supply, and the aetiology of this is not well under stood. As postpartum frequency of milk removal is critical to the establishment of milk production, we compared the early feeding patterns of breastfeeding women with and without GDM. Women with GDM (n = 54) and without GDM (n = 54) provided detailed birth and feeding data within 48 hours of birth and at one and three weeks postpartum and measured their 24 h milk production. Sociodemographic characteristics were similar between groups (p > 0.05), and GDM was associated with an earlier birth gestation (38.5 ± 0.7 vs. 39.5 ± 0.2 weeks, p < 0.001). The median timing of breastfeeding initiation was < 1 h for both groups, yet breastfeeding frequency in the first 24 h was lower in the GDM group (5.9 ± 3.5 vs. 7.8 ± 4.4, p = 0.016). Both in-hospital commercial milk formula supplementation (57% vs. 26%, p < 0.001) and delayed secretory activation beyond day 4 postpartum (32% vs. 7%, p = 0.003) were more prevalent in the GDM group. Combined breastfeeding and breast expression frequencies were similar between groups in the first 24 h (p = 0.48) and at one week (p = 0.46) and three weeks postpartum (p = 0.05). Low milk production (<600 mL/24 h) was more prevalent in the GDM group, i.e., 19/50 (38% compared to those without GDM, i.e., 8/50 (16%), (p = 0.006). Furthermore, four partici pants with GDM had weaned/withdrawn due to low milk supply, i.e., 23/54 (43%). The prevalence of low milk supply, despite frequent breastfeeding and breast expression across the first three weeks postpartum, suggests that endocrine factors may impair the autocrine control of milk production in some women with GDM.

Keywords: gestational diabetes mellitus; breastfeeding; lactation; feeding patterns

Author Contributions: Conceptualization, S.L.P., M.E.W. and D.T.G.; methodology, S.L.P., M.E.W and D.T.G.; software, J.L.M.; validation, S.L.P.; formal analysis, S.L.P.; investigation, S.L.P. and S.A.P. resources, S.A.P. and D.T.G.; data curation, J.L.M.; writing—original draft preparation, S.L.P.; writing— review and editing, D.T.G.; project administration, J.L.M.; funding acquisition, D.T.G. All author have read and agreed to the published version of the manuscript.

Funding: This research was funded by an unrestricted research grant from Medela AG (Switzerland). The funder had no role in the design of the study; in the collection, analyses, or interpretation of data; in the writing of the manuscript; or in the decision to publish the results.

Institutional Review Board Statement: The study was conducted in accordance with the Declaration of Helsinki and approved by The University of Western Australia Human Research Ethics Committee (2019/RA/5/15/1246).

Informed Consent Statement: Informed consent was obtained from all subjects involved in the study.

Data Availability Statement: Restrictions apply to the availability of some or all data generated or analyzed during this study. The corresponding author will upon request detail the restrictions and any conditions under which access to some data may be provided.

Acknowledgments: We thank all study participants for their generous contributions to this study.

Conflicts of Interest: D.T.G. declares past participation in the Scientific Advisory Board of Medela AG. S.L.P., J.L.M., and D.T.G. are supported by an unrestricted research grant from Medela AG administered by The University of Western Australia. The funders had no role in the design of the study; in the collection, analyses, or interpretation of data; in the writing of the manuscript; or in the decision to publish the results. M.E.W. and S.A.P. have no conflicts of interest to declare.

Disclaimer/Publisher's Note: The statements, opinions and data contained in all publications are solely those of the individual author(s) and contributor(s) and not of MDPI and/or the editor(s). MDPI and/or the editor(s) disclaim responsibility for any injury to people or property resulting from any ideas, methods, instructions or products referred to in the content.

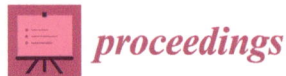 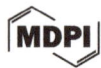

Abstract

Australian Women's Experiences of Returning to Physical Activity in the Year After Birth [†]

Claudia Rich [1,2,3,4], Jacki L. McEachran [1,2,3], Ashleigh H. Warden [1,2,3], Stuart A. Prosser [1,4], Demelza J. Ireland [5], Donna T. Geddes [1,2,3], Zoya Gridneva [1,2,3] and Sharon L. Perrella [1,2,3,4,*]

1. School of Molecular Sciences, The University of Western Australia, Crawley, WA 6009, Australia; claudiaroserich@gmail.com (C.R.); jacki.mceachran@uwa.edu.au (J.L.M.); ashleigh.warden@uwa.edu.au (A.H.W.); stuart@westernobs.com.au (S.A.P.); donna.geddes@uwa.edu.au (D.T.G.); zoya.gridneva@uwa.edu.au (Z.G.)
2. ABREAST Network, Perth, WA 6000, Australia
3. UWA Centre for Human Lactation Research and Translation, Crawley, WA 6009, Australia
4. Western Obstetrics, Balcatta, WA 6021, Australia
5. School of Biomedical Sciences, The University of Western Australia, Crawley, WA 6009, Australia; demelza.ireland@uwa.edu.au
* Correspondence: sharon.perrella@uwa.edu.au
[†] Presented at Australian Breastfeeding + Lactation Research and Science Translation Conference (ABREAST Conference 2024), Perth, Australia, 15 November 2024.

Abstract: While the health advantages of postpartum physical activity are clear, fewer than 25% of Australian women engage in physical activity in the year after giving birth. Physical activity may promote weight loss and a healthier body composition in the months after birth; however, evidence of this is limited. An understanding of identified facilitators and barriers to postpartum physical activity and knowledge of changes in body composition after birth will assist healthcare providers in guiding women on their return to physical activity. The primary aim of this study was to examine Australian women's identified facilitators and barriers to physical activity in the first 12 months postpartum. The secondary aim was to investigate maternal body composition changes between 6–8 weeks and 3–3.5 months postpartum. This study comprised an anonymous online mixed-methods questionnaire and a body composition sub-study. Participants completed an anonymous questionnaire about their pregnancy and birth and their physical activity before and during pregnancy and after birth. Qualitative responses to questions about facilitators and barriers to postpartum physical activity were analysed using content analysis. Sub-study: Women that had given birth within the last 6 weeks were invited to attend study sessions at 6–8 weeks postpartum and then 6 weeks later (3–3.5 months) for anthropometric (weight, height, BMI) and body composition measurements (fat mass, fat-free mass) using a bioelectrical impedance analyser ImpediMed SFB7 (ImpediMed, Brisbane, Queensland, Australia). Participation in physical activity in the previous 7 days and the infant feeding method were recorded at each visit. Survey data of $n = 469$ women were available for analysis. Content analysis of the qualitative data identified the main barriers to physical activity as infant care, timing, and physical limitations. Most survey participants (72%) were active at the time of participation, yet only 23% ($n = 110$) met the postpartum exercise recommendations of 150 minutes/week. The sub-study involving 30 women showed no significant changes in weight ($p = 0.46$), BMI ($p = 0.45$), fat mass ($p = 0.36$), or fat-free mass ($p = 0.23$) between 6–8 weeks and 3–3.5 months postpartum. When compared by breastfeeding status, partially breastfeeding women had a larger magnitude of change in weight (-1.15 ± 1.6 vs. 0.24 ± 1.3 kg, respectively, $p = 0.015$) and BMI (-0.43 ± 0.62 vs. 0.09 ± 0.50 kg/m^2, respectively, $p = 0.016$) than fully breastfeeding women, which may be partly explained by the fat-free mass increase in the latter group (-0.19 ± 2.4

vs. 2.67 ± 5.7 kg, respectively, p = 0.089). At 6–8 weeks postpartum, 45% of participants (n = 14) engaged in at least 150 minutes/week of exercise, with no significant differences in changes in maternal body composition at 3–3.5 months between those meeting the recommendations and those who were not. These findings provide valuable insights that can inform the guidance, support, and education of postpartum women when planning their return to physical activity and form the basis of future studies of exercise and body composition changes in breastfeeding women.

Keywords: physical activity; postpartum; body composition; barriers and facilitators

Author Contributions: Conceptualization, C.R., S.A.P. and S.L.P.; methodology, J.L.M., Z.G. and S.L.P.; formal analysis, C.R., Z.G. and S.L.P.; investigation, C.R.; resources, S.A.P. and D.T.G.; data curation, J.L.M., A.H.W., Z.G. and S.L.P.; writing—original draft preparation, C.R.; writing—review and editing, J.L.M., A.H.W., S.A.P., D.J.I., D.T.G., Z.G. and S.L.P.; supervision, D.J.I., D.T.G., Z.G. and S.L.P.; project administration, J.L.M.; funding acquisition, D.T.G. All authors have read and agreed to the published version of the manuscript.

Funding: This research was funded by an unrestricted research grant from Medela AG (Switzerland). The funder had no role in the design of the study; in the collection, analyses, or interpretation of data; in the writing of the manuscript; or in the decision to publish the results.

Institutional Review Board Statement: This study was conducted in accordance with the Declaration of Helsinki. This study was approved by the Human Research Ethics Committee at The University of Western Australia (2024/ET000140) and conducted in accordance with the relevant guidelines and regulations.

Informed Consent Statement: Informed consent was obtained from all subjects involved in this study.

Data Availability Statement: Restrictions apply to the availability of some or all data generated or analysed during this study. The corresponding author will, upon request, detail the restrictions and any conditions under which access to some data may be provided.

Acknowledgments: We thank all of the participants for their help with this research.

Conflicts of Interest: D.T.G. declares past participation in the Scientific Advisory Board of Medela AG. J.L.M., A.H.W., D.T.G., Z.G. and S.L.P. are supported by an unrestricted research grant from Medela AG, administered by The University of Western Australia. The funder had no role in the design of the study; in the collection, analyses, or interpretation of data; in the writing of the manuscript; or in the decision to publish the results. All other authors declare no conflicts of interest.

Disclaimer/Publisher's Note: The statements, opinions and data contained in all publications are solely those of the individual author(s) and contributor(s) and not of MDPI and/or the editor(s). MDPI and/or the editor(s) disclaim responsibility for any injury to people or property resulting from any ideas, methods, instructions or products referred to in the content.

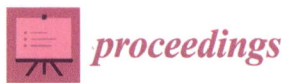

Abstract

Development of the Breastfed Infant Oral Microbiome over the First Two Years of Life in the BLOSOM Cohort [†]

Roaa A. Arishi [1,2,3,4], Ali S. Cheema [5], Ching T. Lai [1,2,3], Matthew S. Payne [6], Donna T. Geddes [1,2,3] and Lisa F. Stinson [1,2,3,*]

[1] School of Molecular Sciences, The University of Western Australia, Perth, WA 6009, Australia; roaa.arishi@research.uwa.edu.au or rarishi@moh.gov.sa (R.A.A.); ching-tat.lai@uwa.edu.au (C.T.L.); donna.geddes@uwa.edu.au (D.T.G.)
[2] ABREAST Network, Perth, WA 6000, Australia
[3] UWA Centre for Human Lactation Research and Translation, Crawley, WA 6009, Australia
[4] Ministry of Health, Riyadh 11176, Saudi Arabia
[5] The Kids Research Institute Australia, Nedlands, WA 6009, Australia; alisadiq.cheema@thekids.org.au
[6] Division of Obstetrics and Gynaecology, The University of Western Australia, Perth, WA 6008, Australia; matthew.payne@uwa.edu.au
* Correspondence: lisa.stinson@uwa.edu.au
[†] Presented at Australian Breastfeeding + Lactation Research and Science Translation Conference (ABREAST Conference 2024), Perth, Australia, 15 November 2024.

Abstract: Acquisition and development of the oral microbiome are dynamic processes that occur during early life. However, data regarding longitudinal assembly and determinants of the infant oral microbiome are sparse. This study aimed to characterise temporal development of the infant oral microbiome during the first two years of life. Infant oral samples (n = 667 samples, 84 infants) were collected at 2–7 days and 1, 2, 3, 4, 5, 6, 9, 12, and 24 months of age using COPAN E-swabs. Bacterial DNA profiles were analysed using full-length 16S rRNA gene sequencing. At 4 months of age, 76.2% of infants were exclusively breastfed, while breastfeeding rates were 83.3% at 6 months and 65.5% at 12 months. The median breastfeeding duration was 12 months (IQR: 3 months). In this cohort, the oral microbiome was dominated by *Streptococcus mitis*, *Gemella haemolysans* and *Rothia mucilaginosa*. Bacterial richness decreased significantly from 1 to 2 months then rose significantly from 12 to 24 months. Shannon diversity increased from 1 week to 1 month and again from 6 to 9 months and 9 to 12 months (all $p \leq 0.04$). Microbiome composition was significantly associated with multiple factors, including pacifier use, intrapartum antibiotic prophylaxis, maternal allergy, pre-pregnancy BMI, siblings, delivery mode, maternal age, pets at home, and birth season (all $p \leq 0.03$). Introduction of solid foods was a significant milestone in oral microbiome development, triggering an increase in bacterial diversity (richness p = 0.0004; Shannon diversity p = 0.0007), a shift in the abundance of seven species, and a change in beta diversity (p = 0.001). These findings underscore how the oral microbiome develops over the first two years of life and highlight the importance of multiple factors, particularly the introduction of solid foods, in shaping the oral microbiome during early life.

Keywords: oral microbiome; temporal; infant diet; breastfeeding; human milk

Author Contributions: Conceptualization, L.F.S., M.S.P. and D.T.G.; methodology, R.A.A. and L.F.S.; formal analysis, R.A.A. and L.F.S.; investigation, R.A.A. and A.S.C.; resources, D.T.G.; data curation, R.A.A.; writing—original draft preparation, R.A.A.; writing—review and editing, R.A.A., L.F.S., M.S.P. and D.T.G.; visualization, R.A.A.; supervision, L.F.S., C.T.L. and D.T.G.; funding acquisition, D.T.G. All authors have read and agreed to the published version of the manuscript.

Funding: This research was funded by an unrestricted research grant from Medela AG (Switzerland), administered by The University of Western Australia. R.A.A. is supported by a PhD postgraduate scholarship from Saudi Arabia. The funders had no role in the design of the study; in the collection, analyses, or interpretation of data; in the writing of the manuscript; or in the decision to publish the results.

Institutional Review Board Statement: The study was conducted in accordance with the Declaration of Helsinki and approved by the Human Research Ethics Committee of The University of Western Australia (RA/4/20/4023).

Informed Consent Statement: Informed consent was obtained from all subjects involved in this study.

Data Availability Statement: Sequence data have been submitted to the NCBI SRA (BioProject Submission: SUB14691294).

Acknowledgments: The authors would like to acknowledge Erika van der Dries for collecting the samples.

Conflicts of Interest: D.T.G. declares participation in the Scientific Advisory Board of Medela AG. C.T.L., L.F.S. and D.T.G. are/were supported by an unrestricted research grant from Medela AG, administered by The University of Western Australia. The funders had no role in the design of the study; in the collection, analyses, or interpretation of data; in the writing of the manuscript; or in the decision to publish the results. All other authors declare no conflicts of interest.

Disclaimer/Publisher's Note: The statements, opinions and data contained in all publications are solely those of the individual author(s) and contributor(s) and not of MDPI and/or the editor(s). MDPI and/or the editor(s) disclaim responsibility for any injury to people or property resulting from any ideas, methods, instructions or products referred to in the content.

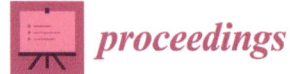

Abstract

Navigating Change: Midwives' Readiness for the Infant Feeding Discussion Page in the West Australian Handheld Pregnancy Record [†]

Shanae K. Paratore [1,2], Kate A. Buchanan [1,2], Sharon L. Perrella [3,4,5] and Sara Bayes [1,2,*]

1. School of Nursing and Midwifery, Edith Cowan University, Joondalup, WA 6027, Australia; s.paratore@ecu.edu.au or shanae.paratore@health.wa.gov.au (S.K.P.); k.buchanan@ecu.edu.au (K.A.B.)
2. Fiona Stanley Hospital, Murdoch, WA 6150, Australia
3. School of Molecular Sciences, The University of Western Australia, Crawley, WA 6009, Australia; sharon.perrella@uwa.edu.au
4. ABREAST Network, Perth, WA 6000, Australia
5. UWA Centre for Human Lactation Research and Translation, Crawley, WA 6009, Australia
* Correspondence: s.bayes@ecu.edu.au; Tel.: +61-6304-2967
† Presented at Australian Breastfeeding + Lactation Research and Science Translation Conference (ABREAST Conference 2024), Perth, Australia, 15 November 2024.

Keywords: midwife; West Australian Handheld Pregnancy Record; midwifery; breastfeeding; prenatal care; antenatal care; Infant Feeding Discussions

Academic Editors: Nicolas L. Taylor and Debbie Palmer

Published: 16 January 2025

Citation: Paratore, S.K.; Buchanan, K.A.; Perrella, S.L.; Bayes, S. Navigating Change: Midwives' Readiness for the Infant Feeding Discussion Page in the West Australian Handheld Pregnancy Record. Proceedings 2025, 112, 19. https://doi.org/10.3390/proceedings112010019

Copyright: © 2025 by the authors. Licensee MDPI, Basel, Switzerland. This article is an open access article distributed under the terms and conditions of the Creative Commons Attribution (CC BY) license (https://creativecommons.org/licenses/by/4.0/).

In Western Australia (WA), women accessing public maternity care services are given a West Australian Handheld Pregnancy Record (WAHPR) booklet that includes pages where health care professionals record the pregnancy care and education provided. The latest revision of the booklet, implemented in November 2023, included a new "Infant Feeding Discussion" page that requires the sharing of infant feeding information at six antenatal time points and an updated breastfeeding information page where women are asked to identify lactation risk factors such as previous breast/nipple surgery or piercing, diabetes or a previous difficult breastfeeding experience, and invited to discuss these with their midwife, lactation consultant or peer supporter. In WA, it is midwives who predominantly provide antenatal information and education on infant feeding matters. Women and other birthing people's infant feeding decisions are strongly influenced by the "preference, advice and practice" of the health professionals they encounter [1], so research to explore those phenomena is appropriate. Additionally, the WAHPR represents a practice change, and it is well known that in healthcare, myriad "context readiness" challenges can hinder the successful implementation of changes such as this [2]. These challenges broadly exist at the micro- (individual), meso- (group), and macro- (wider institutional) levels [3].

The aim of this study was to understand the attitudes and readiness of midwives working in WA with pregnant women to lead the discussions about infant feeding and breastfeeding required of them in the new WAHPR. A convergent mixed methods design was employed to determine the responses of WA-based midwives who regularly use the WAHPR when providing antenatal care. Recruitment was conducted through social media, specifically Facebook community pages for WA midwives and the Australian College of Midwives community, with a direct link to an electronic survey. Participants provided informed consent before completing a 12-item online anonymous survey with quantitative and qualitative items that took <20 min to complete.

Responses were received from n = 23 midwives, of which 15 (65%) had $\geq$5 years of midwifery experience. Ten (43%) reported that breastfeeding education is a key part of their role, and eighteen (78%) indicated that this was a very important part of their role. In relation to the WAHPR "Infant Feeding Discussion" and "Breastfeeding Information" pages ten (43%) of midwives felt quite confident to have these discussions, whilst only seven (30%) felt extremely confident. Of the 17 participants who provided qualitative feedback, 5 (29%) indicated that a barrier to adequate discussion was antenatal appointment time constraints. Of those who did not feel confident in conducting infant feeding discussions, the need for further training in breastfeeding was a commonly cited theme. Twenty (86%) midwives felt some professional development would be helpful, allowing them to work with the Infant Feeding Discussion and Breastfeeding Information Pages in the WAHPR. Fourteen (60%) midwives would prefer the format of this professional development to be a mix of some taught content and some self-directed study, whilst thirteen (56%) preferred self-directed study.

Midwives value the importance of infant feeding discussions and generally feel confident but face challenges such as time constraints and lack of training related to using the new Infant Feeding Discussions protocol. Most supported additional professional development, favoring a combination of taught and self-directed learning to enhance confidence and effectiveness in using the new WAHPR infant feeding and breastfeeding pages. The study findings support the development of flexible, professional development programs, addressing time constraints, and providing updated resources. Further study is required to monitor the integration of the WAHPR's Infant Feeding and Breastfeeding Information pages and suggested changes to enhance midwives' confidence and effectiveness in antenatal care.

Author Contributions: Conceptualization, S.L.P. and S.B.; methodology, S.K.P., K.A.B., S.L.P. and S.B.; software, S.K.P. and S.B.; formal analysis, S.K.P. and S.L.P.; investigation, S.K.P., K.A.B., S.L.P. and S.B.; resources, S.B.; data curation, S.B.; writing—original draft preparation, S.L.P. and S.K.P.; writing—review and editing, K.A.B. and S.B.; supervision, K.A.B. and S.B.; project administration, S.K.P.; funding acquisition, S.B. All authors have read and agreed to the published version of the manuscript.

Funding: This research was funded by Edith Cowan University. S.L.P. is supported by an unrestricted research grant from Medela AG, administered by The University of Western Australia. The funders had no role in the design of the study; in the collection, analyses, or interpretation of data; in the writing of the manuscript; or in the decision to publish the results.

Institutional Review Board Statement: The study was conducted in accordance with the Declaration of Helsinki. The study was approved by the Human Research Ethics Committee at Edith Cowan University (2023-04947-PARATORE), with recognition of prior ethics approval provided by The University of Western Australia, and conducted in accordance with the relevant guidelines and regulations.

Informed Consent Statement: Informed consent was obtained from all subjects involved in the study.

Data Availability Statement: Restrictions apply to the availability of some, or all data generated or analyzed during this study. The corresponding author will, on request, detail the restrictions and any conditions under which access to some data may be provided.

Acknowledgments: We thank all of the participants for their help with this research.

Conflicts of Interest: S.L.P. is supported by an unrestricted research grant from Medela AG, administered by The University of Western Australia. The funder had no role in the design of the study; in the collection, analysis, or interpretation of data; in the writing of the manuscript; or in the decision to publish the results. All other authors declare no conflicts of interest.

References

1. Matriano, M.G.; Ivers, R.; Meedya, S. Factors that influence women's decision on infant feeding: An integrative review. *Women Birth* **2022**, *35*, 430–439. [CrossRef] [PubMed]
2. Nilsen, P.; Bernhardsson, S. Context matters in implementation science: A scoping review of determinant frameworks that describe contextual determinants for implementation outcomes. *BMC Health Serv. Res.* **2019**, *19*, 1–21. [CrossRef] [PubMed]
3. Squires, J.E.; Graham, I.D.; Santos, W.J.; Hutchinson, A.M.; ICON Team. The Implementation in Context (ICON) Framework: A meta-framework of context domains, attributes and features in healthcare. *Health Res. Policy Syst.* **2023**, *21*, 81. [CrossRef] [PubMed]

Disclaimer/Publisher's Note: The statements, opinions and data contained in all publications are solely those of the individual author(s) and contributor(s) and not of MDPI and/or the editor(s). MDPI and/or the editor(s) disclaim responsibility for any injury to people or property resulting from any ideas, methods, instructions or products referred to in the content.

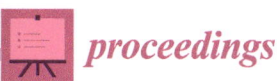

Abstract

Breastfeeding Characteristics Are Associated with Minor Changes in the Human Milk Microbiome [†]

Ruomei Xu [1,2,3], Mark P. Nicol [2,4], Ali S. Cheema [5], Jacki L. McEachran [1,2,3], Sharon L. Perrella [1,2,3], Zoya Gridneva [1,2,3], Donna T. Geddes [1,2,3] and Lisa F. Stinson [1,2,3,*]

1. School of Molecular Sciences, The University of Western Australia, Crawley, WA 6009, Australia; ruomei.xu@research.uwa.edu.au (R.X.); jacki.mceachran@uwa.edu.au (J.L.M.); sharon.perrella@uwa.edu.au (S.L.P.); zoya.gridneva@uwa.edu.au (Z.G.); donna.geddes@uwa.edu.au (D.T.G.)
2. UWA Centre for Human Lactation Research and Translation, Crawley, WA 6009, Australia; mark.nicol@uwa.edu.au
3. ABREAST Network, Perth, WA 6000, Australia
4. School of Biomedical Sciences, The University of Western Australia, Crawley, WA 6009, Australia
5. The Kids Research Institute Australia, Nedlands, WA 6009, Australia; alisadiq.cheema@telethonkids.org.au
* Correspondence: lisa.stinson@uwa.edu.au; Tel.: +61-8-6488-3200
† Presented at Australian Breastfeeding + Lactation Research and Science Translation Conference (ABREAST Conference 2024), Perth, Australia, 15 November 2024.

Keywords: human milk; microbiome; breastfeeding characteristics; milk production; infant

Human milk has a microbiome that contains a wide variety of typical oral and skin bacteria, suggesting that the bacterial communities in the infant oral cavity and maternal skin contribute to the development of the human milk microbiome [1–3]. It is hypothesised that breastfeeding characteristics, such as feeding frequencies, total 24 h breastfeeding duration and breast pump use, could lead to different levels of exposure to oral and skin bacteria and subsequently altered bacterial profiles in human milk. In order to investigate the associations between breastfeeding characteristics and the human milk microbiome, this study analysed milk samples collected from 57 healthy lactating women at 3 months postpartum by full-length 16S rRNA gene sequencing. The results showed that breastfeeding characteristics were associated with neither Shannon diversity nor richness of the human milk microbiome. Total 24 h breastfeeding duration, however, was positively associated with *Streptococcus salivarius* (0.013 ± 0.006, $p = 0.035$). Mothers with normal milk production (≥600 mL/24 h) harboured less *Streptococcus parasanguinis* (−0.007 ± 0.003, $p = 0.035$) and *Veillonella* sp. (−0.008 ± 0.003, $p = 0.011$) in the milk. Breastfeeding frequency was positively associated with *Pseudomonas* sp. (0.204 ± 0.098, $p = 0.042$). In conclusion, total 24 h breastfeeding duration, breastfeeding frequency and 24 h milk production were associated with specific bacterial species in human milk.

Author Contributions: Conceptualization, L.F.S., M.P.N. and D.T.G.; methodology, L.F.S.; formal analysis, R.X. and L.F.S.; investigation, R.X. and A.S.C.; resources, D.T.G.; data curation, Z.G., S.L.P., J.L.M. and R.X.; writing—original draft preparation, R.X.; writing—review and editing, M.P.N., L.F.S., A.S.C., J.L.M., Z.G., S.L.P. and D.T.G.; visualization, R.X.; supervision, L.F.S., D.T.G. and M.P.N.; funding acquisition, D.T.G. All authors have read and agreed to the published version of the manuscript.

Funding: This research is funded by an unrestricted research grant from Medela AG (Switzerland).

Institutional Review Board Statement: The study was conducted in accordance with the Declaration of Helsinki and approved by the Human Research Ethics Committee of The University of Western Australia (RA/4/20/4023).

Informed Consent Statement: Informed consent was obtained from all subjects involved in the study.

Data Availability Statement: Sequence data have been submitted to the NCBI SRA (BioProject Submission: SUB13951443).

Acknowledgments: The authors would like to acknowledge Erika van den Dries for collecting the samples and Matthew Payne for the use of his laboratory space and equipment.

Conflicts of Interest: D.T.G. declares participation in the Scientific Advisory Board of Medela AG. D.T.G., J.L.M., Z.G. and L.F.S. receive a salary from an unrestricted research grant from Medela AG administered by The University of Western Australia. The funders had no role in the design of the study; in the collection, analyses, or interpretation of data; in the writing of the manuscript; or in the decision to publish the results. M.P.N. and A.S.C. declare no conflicts of interest.

References

1. Cheema, A.S.; Trevenen, M.L.; Turlach, B.A.; Furst, A.J.; Roman, A.S.; Bode, L.; Gridneva, Z.; Lai, C.T.; Stinson, L.F.; Payne, M.S.; et al. Exclusively Breastfed Infant Microbiota Develops over Time and Is Associated with Human Milk Oligosaccharide Intakes. *Int. J. Mol. Sci.* **2022**, *23*, 2804. [CrossRef]
2. Moossavi, S.; Sepehri, S.; Robertson, B.; Bode, L.; Goruk, S.; Field, C.J.; Lix, L.M.; de Souza, R.J.; Becker, A.B.; Mandhane, P.J.; et al. Composition and variation of the human milk microbiota are influenced by maternal and early-life factors. *Cell Host Microbe* **2019**, *25*, 324–335.e4. [CrossRef] [PubMed]
3. Ramsay, D.T.; Kent, J.C.; Owens, R.A.; Hartmann, P.E. Ultrasound imaging of milk ejection in the breast of lactating women. *Pediatrics* **2004**, *113*, 361–367. [CrossRef] [PubMed]

Disclaimer/Publisher's Note: The statements, opinions and data contained in all publications are solely those of the individual author(s) and contributor(s) and not of MDPI and/or the editor(s). MDPI and/or the editor(s) disclaim responsibility for any injury to people or property resulting from any ideas, methods, instructions or products referred to in the content.

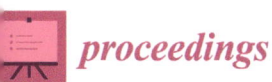

Abstract

Women's Experiences of Establishing Breastfeeding After Assisted and Unassisted Vaginal Birth [†]

Evangeline G. Bevan [1,2,3,4], Jacki L. McEachran [1,2,3], Demelza J. Ireland [4], Stuart A. Prosser [1,5], Donna T. Geddes [1,2,3] and Sharon L. Perrella [1,2,3,5,*]

1 School of Molecular Sciences, The University of Western Australia, Crawley, WA 6009, Australia; jacki.mceachran@uwa.edu.au (J.L.M.); stuart@westernobs.com.au (S.A.P.); donna.geddes@uwa.edu.au (D.T.G.)
2 ABREAST Network, Perth, WA 6000, Australia
3 UWA Centre for Human Lactation Research and Translation, Crawley, WA 6009, Australia
4 School of Biomedical Sciences, The University of Western Australia, Crawley, WA 6009, Australia; demelza.ireland@uwa.edu.au
5 Western Obstetrics, Balcatta, WA 6021, Australia
* Correspondence: sharon.perrella@uwa.edu.au
† Presented at Australian Breastfeeding + Lactation Research and Science Translation Conference (ABREAST Conference 2024), Perth, Australia, 15 November 2024.

Abstract: Vacuum-assisted and forceps-assisted vaginal births are associated with higher rates of formula supplementation and shorter breastfeeding duration compared to unassisted vaginal births; however, the reasons for this are unclear. Factors such as maternal knowledge, partner support, and parity significantly influence breastfeeding initiation and duration. The prevalence of perineal trauma, neonatal and maternal birth complications, and decreased birth satisfaction is higher after assisted births and may also impact breastfeeding outcomes. Given the limited research on the specific effects of different vaginal birth modes on breastfeeding, this study aimed to examine women's experiences of establishing breastfeeding after unassisted, vacuum-assisted, and forceps-assisted vaginal birth. A mixed-methods study design was employed using an anonymous online questionnaire, which included binary, multiple choice, and open-ended questions, and Likert scale items. Using social media, we recruited Australian women who had an unassisted, vacuum-assisted, or forceps-assisted birth within the last year. Details of participant demographics, breastfeeding history, initiation and establishment, postpartum mobility, and pain ratings were recorded. Additionally, qualitative data on postpartum recovery and breastfeeding support were analysed using an inductive thematic analysis framework. A total of 565 women were recruited between May and June 2024, of which 488 responses were retained for analysis. Thematic analysis of the qualitative responses identified four central themes that defined women's experiences of establishing breastfeeding and were similar between unassisted or assisted vaginal birth modes: Experience of Care, Environment, Expectations, and Health Complications. A range of both positive and negative experiences of breastfeeding support, environmental factors, and expectations of the realities of breastfeeding impacted women's experiences. For many women, various maternal and/or newborn health issues, nipple pain, and latching difficulties made breastfeeding more difficult. Commercial milk formula supplementation during the hospital stay was more prevalent after a forceps-assisted birth when compared to unassisted vaginal birth (41% vs. 17%, respectively; $p < 0.001$). Further, during the first two weeks at home, commercial milk formula supplementation was more prevalent after both forceps-assisted (26%) and vacuum-assisted (23%) births than after unassisted vaginal birth (8%, $p < 0.001$). Pain ratings in the early days following birth and in the first two weeks at home were significantly higher for the forceps-assisted group than for the other vaginal birth modes ($p \leq 0.005$).

Women that had an unassisted vaginal birth with an intact perineum had the lowest pain ratings in the early days and weeks after birth, while pain ratings were similar between women that had a vacuum-assisted birth and those who had an unassisted vaginal birth with a perineal tear or episiotomy ($p = 0.05$). Early commercial milk formula supplementation is associated with shorter breastfeeding duration, while postpartum pain is known to impede maternal mobility and may partially inhibit the milk ejection reflex, potentially negatively impacting breastfeeding and increasing formula use. Therefore, women who have an instrumental assisted vaginal birth, particularly those who have a forceps-assisted birth, are at greater risk of suboptimal breastfeeding outcomes including short durations of exclusive and any breastfeeding. Improvements to early postpartum pain management, breastfeeding education, and the judicious use of commercial milk formula may improve breastfeeding and subsequent maternal and health outcomes after instrument-assisted vaginal birth.

Keywords: breast feeding; exclusive breastfeeding; postpartum; postnatal care; obstetrical forceps; vacuum extraction; obstetrical; episiotomy; pelvic floor; pelvic pain

---

Author Contributions: Conceptualization, D.T.G. and S.L.P.; methodology, E.G.B., J.L.M., S.A.P. and S.L.P.; formal analysis, E.G.B. and S.L.P.; investigation, E.G.B.; resources, D.T.G.; data curation, J.L.M. and S.L.P.; writing—original draft preparation, E.G.B.; writing—review and editing, J.L.M., D.J.I., S.A.P., D.T.G. and S.L.P.; supervision, D.J.I., D.T.G. and S.L.P.; project administration, J.L.M.; funding acquisition, D.T.G. All authors have read and agreed to the published version of the manuscript.

Funding: This research was funded by an unrestricted research grant from Medela AG (Switzerland). The funder had no role in the design of the study; in the collection, analyses, or interpretation of data; in the writing of the manuscript; or in the decision to publish the results.

Institutional Review Board Statement: The study was conducted in accordance with the Declaration of Helsinki. The study was approved by the Human Research Ethics Committee at The University of Western Australia (2024/ET000323) and conducted in accordance with the relevant guidelines and regulations.

Informed Consent Statement: Informed consent was obtained from all subjects involved in the study.

Data Availability Statement: Restrictions apply to the availability of some or all data generated or analyzed during this study. The corresponding author will on request detail the restrictions and any conditions under which access to some data may be provided.

Acknowledgments: We thank all of the participants for help with this research.

Conflicts of Interest: D.T.G. declares past participation in the Scientific Advisory Board of Medela AG. J.L.M., D.T.G. and S.L.P. are supported by an unrestricted research grant from Medela AG administered by The University of Western Australia. The funder had no role in the design of the study; in the collection, analyses, or interpretation of data; in the writing of the manuscript; or in the decision to publish the results. All other authors declare no conflicts of interest.

Disclaimer/Publisher's Note: The statements, opinions and data contained in all publications are solely those of the individual author(s) and contributor(s) and not of MDPI and/or the editor(s). MDPI and/or the editor(s) disclaim responsibility for any injury to people or property resulting from any ideas, methods, instructions or products referred to in the content.

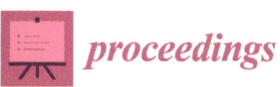

Abstract

Nanoscale Imaging of Human Milk Cells [†]

Qiongxiang Lin [1,2], Sharon L. Perrella [1,3,4], Ashleigh H. Warden [1,3,4], Cameron W. Evans [1,2], Donna T. Geddes [1,2,3,4], Leon R. Mitoulas [1,2,5], Haibo Jiang [1,2,6], Kai Chen [2,7] and Killugudi Swaminatha Iyer [1,2,*]

1. School of Molecular Sciences, The University of Western Australia, Crawley, WA 6009, Australia; 23859469@student.uwa.edu.au (Q.L.); sharon.perrella@uwa.edu.au (S.L.P.); ashleigh.warden@uwa.edu.au (A.H.W.); cameron.evans@uwa.edu.au (C.W.E.); donna.geddes@uwa.edu.au (D.T.G.); leon.mitoulas@medela.com (L.R.M.); haibo.jiang@uwa.edu.au (H.J.)
2. ARC Training Centre for Next-Gen in Biomedical Analysis, School of Molecular Sciences, The University of Western Australia, Perth, WA 6009, Australia; kai.chen@uwa.edu.au
3. ABREAST Network, Perth, WA 6000, Australia
4. UWA Centre for Human Lactation Research and Translation, Crawley, WA 6009, Australia
5. Medela AG, ZUG 6340 Baar, Switzerland
6. Department of Chemistry, The University of Hong Kong, Pok Fu Lam, Hong Kong 999077, China
7. School of Biomedical Sciences, The University of Western Australia, Crawley, WA 6009, Australia
* Correspondence: swaminatha.iyer@uwa.edu.au
† Presented at Australian Breastfeeding + Lactation Research and Science Translation Conference (ABREAST Conference 2024), Perth, Australia, 15 November 2024.

Abstract: Human milk is a complex biofluid containing a diverse array of cells crucial for infant health. Despite their importance, our understanding of these cells remains incomplete due to technical challenges. To fully comprehend human milk cells, high-resolution imaging technologies that can directly measure biological processes are required. We have developed a specialized imaging platform combining light and electron microscopy for human milk cell imaging. To identify different cell types, human milk cells were first stained with several specific cell markers (e.g., EpCAM and MUC1 for lactocytes, CD16 and CD66b for neutrophils, and HLA-DR and CD68 for macrophages) prior to light (confocal) microscopy. Following this, the same cells were processed with osmium staining, resin embedding, and sectioning for electron microscopy, allowing us to observe ultrastructural details. Our imaging workflow has enabled nanoscale visualization of human milk cells, resulting in a first-of-its-kind comprehensive database profiling the organelle-level ultrastructure of different cell types present in human milk. The cells in the human milk are highly heterogenous, featuring a large proportion of lactocytes and lipid droplets, binucleated lactocytes, neutrophil aggregation, neutrophil extracellular traps, dendritic cells/macrophages with bacteria, and immunophagocytosis. This study provides valuable cellular insights contributing to a deeper understanding of human milk biology.

Keywords: human milk cells; nanoscale imaging; organelle-level ultrastructure; lactocytes; neutrophils; dendritic cells: macrophages; correlatively light–electron microscopy

Author Contributions: Conceptualization, K.S.I., K.C. and H.J.; methodology, Q.L., K.S.I., K.C., H.J., C.W.E., D.T.G., S.L.P. and A.H.W.; formal analysis, Q.L. and K.C.; investigation, A.H.W. and S.L.P.; resources, K.S.I., D.T.G. and L.R.M.; writing—original draft preparation, Q.L.; writing—review and editing, K.S.I., K.C., H.J., C.W.E., D.T.G., L.R.M., S.L.P. and A.H.W.; supervision, C.W.E. and K.S.I.; funding acquisition, K.S.I. All authors have read and agreed to the published version of the manuscript.

Funding: This research was funded by the Australian Research Council (ARC) (Project ID: IC210100056). Q.L. is supported by the Research Training Program Fees Offset Scholarship and ARC On-Water Electrochemistry HDR Scholarship. D.T.G., S.L.P., and A.H.W. are supported by an unrestricted research grant from Medela AG (Switzerland), administered by The University of Western Australia. L.R.M. is supported by Medela AG. The funders had no role in the design of the study; in the collection, analyses, or interpretation of data; in the writing of the manuscript; or in the decision to publish the results.

Institutional Review Board Statement: The study was conducted in accordance with the Declaration of Helsinki and approved by the UWA Human Research Ethics Committee (2019/RA/4/20/6498; the date of approval 21/02/2024).

Informed Consent Statement: Informed consent was obtained from all participants involved in the study.

Acknowledgments: We thank all the participants who donated breast milk for the study.

Conflicts of Interest: D.T.G. declares past participation in the Scientific Advisory Board of Medela. AG. D.T.G., S.L.P. and A.H.W. are supported by an unrestricted research grant from Medela AG, administered by The University of Western Australia. L.R.M. is supported by Medela AG. The funder had no role in the design of the study; in the collection, analyses, or interpretation of data; in the writing of the manuscript; or in the decision to publish the results. All other authors declare no conflicts of interest.

Disclaimer/Publisher's Note: The statements, opinions and data contained in all publications are solely those of the individual author(s) and contributor(s) and not of MDPI and/or the editor(s). MDPI and/or the editor(s) disclaim responsibility for any injury to people or property resulting from any ideas, methods, instructions or products referred to in the content.

MDPI AG
Grosspeteranlage 5
4052 Basel
Switzerland
Tel.: +41 61 683 77 34

Proceedings Editorial Office
E-mail: proceedings@mdpi.com
www.mdpi.com/journal/proceedings

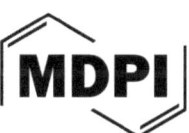

Disclaimer/Publisher's Note: The title and front matter of this reprint are at the discretion of the Volume Editors. The publisher is not responsible for their content or any associated concerns. The statements, opinions and data contained in all individual articles are solely those of the individual Editors and contributors and not of MDPI. MDPI disclaims responsibility for any injury to people or property resulting from any ideas, methods, instructions or products referred to in the content.

www.ingramcontent.com/pod-product-compliance
Lightning Source LLC
LaVergne TN
LVHW072252110526
838202LV00106B/2616